PRAISE FOR

THE PATIENT'S SURVIVAL GUIDE

"It is common sense to assume that improvements in population health are a direct consequence of the advances of diagnosis and treatment for which the healthcare system is quick to take credit. But a great many of the putative advances have withstood scientific scrutiny poorly, if at all. There has been a choir singing that truth for some time. Ed Morgan is contributing his voice to that choir. He brings a keen perspective tempered by a life course devoted to caring about those in need. *The Patient's Survival Guide* is a clarion call. Perhaps this is the voice that will fill the pews."

—NORTIN M HADLER, MD, MACP, MACR, FACOEM

"Ed Morgan presents a set of facts, arguments, and warnings we all need to heed. With overtreatment and medical mistakes now the third leading cause of death in the U.S., we need to ask the tough questions of our doctors before agreeing to surgery, long-term medications and other treatments. With a commitment to lifestyle change, Ed enables his readers to recognize that you must be in charge of your health."

—ROBERT DOLL, CHIEF INVESTMENT OFFICER,
CROSSMARK GLOBAL INVESTMENTS

the
PATIENT'S
SURVIVAL GUIDE

the
PATIENT'S
SURVIVAL GUIDE

SEVEN KEY QUESTIONS for
NAVIGATING THE MEDICAL MAZE

EDWARD H. MORGAN JR.

BEAUFORT
BOOKS

The PATIENT'S SURVIVAL GUIDE

First Edition

Copyright 2022 Edward H. Morgan Jr.

This book is not intended as a substitute for the medical advice of physicians. The reader should consult a physician in matters relating to his/her health and particularly with respect to any symptoms that may require diagnosis or medical attention.

Paperback ISBN: 9780825309885

Ebook ISBN: 9780825308673

For inquiries about volume orders, please contact:

Beaufort Books, 27 West 20th Street, Suite 1103, New York, NY 10011

sales@beaufortbooks.com

Published in the United States by Beaufort Books

www.beaufortbooks.com

Distributed by Midpoint Trade Books

a division of Independent Publisher Group

www.ipgbook.com

Book designed by Mark Karis

Printed in the United States of America

TO DAD

Who got caught in unwise treatment and died before his time

CONTENTS

PART III: NEW WAYS OF THINKING

PROLOGUE

It's a curious thing, when you're in your mid-seventies, and you realize you have a book in you.

You push it aside; it comes back. Your friends are polite, too polite to tell you you're totally unqualified to write it.

You have a fifty-year marriage to celebrate; you have sons and grandchildren to attend to. People want to talk to you about leadership and board governance.

Yet, this is the junkyard dog with its teeth in your ankle. It won't let go. Stories come to you; they fall in your lap. People tell you their scary medical stories.

And then you realize you see their stories through a different lens than they do. And that you've seen medical stories through a different lens for decades. You saw what was happening to your dad, but you were unable to save him from an early death. But you probably saved your wife from an early demise, and you did save yourself from becoming a heart patient instead of a well person.

You realize that you've got to try to help your family see their medical experiences through a different lens—a lens of wisdom and independent thinking—or else they could die early. You know that the US medical system can be dangerous to your health, and will be, if you use it without discretion and let it over-diagnose you, overtreat you, and shorten your life.

I've had a few insights during my career that stretched the rubber band of conventionality far enough to create disbelief. When I proposed as CEO that the Bowery Mission could adopt a New York fundraising "art form" called a gala to create a million-dollar event for a little religious charity, people were skeptical. But they were willing to listen—and I made it happen.

But when you propose that in certain circumstances you need to go against your doctor's sincere advice, this stretches the rubber band until it breaks, doesn't it? If you can't trust your own doctor, where can you go? Do you know more than he or she does? Preposterous.

So the ideas in this book are a hard sell. The idea that the third leading cause of death in the US might be iatrogenic (medically caused) is hard to wrap your head around. It produces a negative visceral reaction. I recognize that this guide starts with a premise altogether foreign to most people—so foreign it's like changing political parties. If you are not ready to tackle such a perspective-changing topic, I understand. And if you've never had a negative encounter with big medicine, I don't consider you a likely prospect, unless you already possess generic wisdom.

But remember this. I set out to write an indictment of big medicine in this country. But then I realized that indictment has already been written more than thirty times in the last twenty years or so by highly qualified physicians, passionate reformers, and grieving parents of children. They all took on the establishment and lost. Many are cited here.

So I'm writing a wisdom guide, not a blockbuster.

My hope is that you, the reader, will make the huge leap from the comfort of complete medical compliance to teamwork with your doctor to discover the truth and live to a ripe old age.

AUTHOR'S NOTE

This book offers a personal perspective on healthcare as an individual contributor, not a health professional. The health and medical information herein should not be construed as medical advice and should be used to supplement, not replace, the advice of your physician or another trained health professional. Both the publisher and I disclaim liability for any medical outcomes that may occur as a result of applying the principles suggested in this book. This book has been carefully and independently fact checked. However, any remaining errors, misattributions, inaccuracies, or other defects are my responsibility alone.

FOREWORD

by DR. NORTIN HADLER

We are bombarded with mixed medical messages these days—news of dire threats to our health and news of medical miracles that are available or will be soon. There is no doubt that some threats are real and that some medical advances are substantive. But these mixed messages have created a sense of unease in our society that even permeates into the center of the medical profession where I have served for decades.

The medical students I have taught, the distinguished colleagues I have worked with, and most of all, the patients I was pledged to help all sense medicine is different than it used to be, and not all of the change is good.

Mixed messaging causes cognitive dissonance, escalates uncertainty, provokes anxiety, and thwarts rational decision making. We've been living with a degree of health insecurity that has escalated since the mid-twentieth century despite dramatic improvements in population health.

It is common sense to assume the improvement in population health is a direct consequence of the advances in diagnosis and treatment for which the health care system and healthcare industry are quick to take credit. I am no Luddite; there have been important advances. But a great many of the putative advances have withstood scientific scrutiny poorly, if at all. There has been a choir singing that truth for some time.

The same choir urges any person who chooses to be a patient to feel empowered to ask for detailed assurance that any medical or surgical intervention offers enough likelihood of benefit so that the patient can discount potential downsides. This is called informed medical decision making. The patient defines risk tolerance. This is a collaboration between a physician who informs and a patient who feels empowered. Ed Morgan is contributing his voice to this choir. He brings a keen perspective tempered by a life-course devoted to caring about those in need. *The Patient Survival Guide* is a clarion call. Perhaps this is the voice that will fill the pews.

—**NORTIN M. HADLER, MD, MACP, MACR, FACOEM** IS PROFESSOR OF MEDICINE, EMERITUS AT THE UNIVERSITY OF NORTH CAROLINA AT CHAPEL HILL AND AUTHOR OF NUMEROUS BOOKS INCLUDING *WORRIED SICK: A PRESCRIPTION FOR HEALTH IN AN OVERTREATED AMERICA*, AND *THE LAST WELL PERSON: HOW TO STAY WELL DESPITE THE HEALTHCARE SYSTEM.*

PREFACE

In a sense, this guide has been about seventy years in the making. I had an early experience of medically induced complications (now called iatrogenic disease) at a time when they were relatively rare. You might even say I was a "drug-reaction pioneer."

In 1949, when I was in second grade in Springfield, Delaware County, Pennsylvania, our family doctor prescribed a sulfonamide antibiotic, one of the earliest "miracle" antibiotics, for a common childhood infection.

After a few days on this drug, this seven-year-old came down with acute nephritis (kidney inflammation). Renal function dropped, edema set in, and I ended up in Philadelphia Osteopathic Hospital while doctors figured out what to do.

There was actually very little to do at the time except pray, hydrate, avoid salt (Epsom salts instead), and rest. Lots of rest. In fact, it was deemed I should "rest" for a whole year. So I spent all of third grade resting on a chaise longue and reading. (I'm still not good at sports!)

But the upsides of that year were my full recovery, my later interest in iatrogenic matters, and the development of my reading and academic ability. I had finished second grade reading just at grade level but finished third grade reading at the tenth-grade level—with a vocabulary to match.

So this unfortunate incident has helped me all my life. Being a voracious reader has helped me through my nineteen years as a communicator for General Electric senior executives, twenty-two years as CEO of New York's Bowery Mission, and now, finally, in my own consulting practice on leadership. And now it is helping me come full circle with this guide.

Throughout my life, I have kept myself informed not only on the amazing and lifesaving explosion of medical knowledge, treatments, and technology, but also on the more ominous development of aggressive Big Pharma, risky diagnostics, low productivity mass screenings, and aggressive protocols substituted for clinical judgment. These profit-fueled and patient-endangering practices have grown into a monster—a national emergency that has become the third leading cause of death in America. More on that in the next chapter.

There are a few courageous doctors out there talking about these things, like the more than thirty authors in the "Further Reading" section. But they mostly get no mainstream media attention. The electronic media, with the commendable exception of the focus on the opioid crisis, seem uninterested in stories on our broken medical system and its thousands of unnecessary deaths, stories that will cross their Big Pharma sponsors; instead they extol high-tech medical breakthroughs that benefit very few and feature milquetoast advice for better health. The print media have done somewhat better, but to little effect, and the younger generation consumes mostly electronic media.

Hence, I decided to get practical and construct this guide with the hope that it will help prevent medical tragedies and extend a friend or a family member's longevity. That's why I'm writing.

The need for this kind of skeptical wisdom has risen exponentially in the past two decades. Overtreatment and medical mistakes have multiplied into the premature deaths of hundreds of thousands. We explain how in chapter 1. A couple of examples close to home:

My father died in 1991 at seventy-five years of age of metastatic prostate cancer. I show in this guide how it is probable that he didn't need to die that young.

In 1999, my wife was diagnosed with stage 1 breast cancer, had a lumpectomy, some local radiation, and no chemotherapy. Two hospitals, including one of the leading cancer hospitals in the nation, recommended a full round of chemotherapy, even though there was no lymph node involvement. When I asked for any studies on five-year recurrence of stage 1 breast cancer, with or without chemotherapy, first there were raised eyebrows that I would question their clinical judgment and established protocols. Second, I was told there were no such studies. Finally, a small study was proffered, which showed a 2% absolute difference in recurrence, which is not statistically significant in a study that small. When asked why they would not save "the big guns" for when and if the cancer returned and help keep my wife's immune system intact, there was further patronizing talk—talk of killing every last remaining cancer cell—a totally improbable and unverifiable goal. We walked. Twenty-one years later there has been no recurrence.

One more story ripened my conviction that I should write about this. I had my own brush with becoming a heart patient. In October of 2018, I noticed some shortness of breath and angina-like symptoms when taking the subway stairs quickly in New York City, as I usually do. Chest discomfort during exercise is never a good thing, although it can have multiple causes, as I was about to learn. I saw our family physician, who praised me for coming in and sent me right over to an interventional cardiologist. I suggested a non-invasive stress test on a treadmill with an echocardiogram as a first step, and he agreed. But the stress test results were not "normal" and led to a recommendation for angiography to see the extent of any artery blockages. The possibility of implanting a stent was mentioned.

A caution light went on in my head, and I told him we would get back to him. The next few days of research were eye-opening. I had a cardiologist friend in New York read the echocardiogram and EKG and review the notes as a first step.

And in the following nights, I googled "unnecessary heart stents" and was literally knocked back by page after page of results, both from popular sources like the *New York Times* and from peer-reviewed journals. The upshot, as reported later in this book: there's a $2.9 billion heart stent industry in North America[1] with a million angioplasty procedures performed in 2019[2]—life-saving procedures if performed during heart attacks but apparently of zero worth in reducing mortality if used prophylactically. In addition, the blood thinners required after implantation have caused thousands of complications.

I declined the procedure, took statins and a baby aspirin for a few months, added cardio-exercises three times a week, and lowered my sugar intake. One year later, the symptoms are gone. This does not mean that anyone should ignore chest pain or refuse all suggested interventions. It does mean that we should proceed with caution and wisdom when interventional cardiology is recommended.

I am well aware that medical harm has been going on since the time of Hippocrates and his famous admonition to physicians to "first do no harm." And I am also aware that medical harm has been going on in this country since George Washington's physicians bled him profusely during his final illness. But I think we should all be shocked by how the cautious approach of the Hippocratic oath that all new doctors take has been replaced by the notion that an aggressive medical approach is almost always the best for the patient and certainly for the doctor in this litigious climate. The harvest of this notion is detailed in the next chapter.

I realize that many people will be skeptical. Most people believe that medical harm has declined as ignorance-based treatments have disappeared. Would that it was so! To the contrary, medical harm has ballooned into an epidemic as new dimensions of unintended consequences take over medicine—rooted in overdiagnosis, overtreatment, flawed pharmaceutical studies, and doctors worried about lawsuits. In today's American medical system, many incentives for health care providers are misaligned with the interests of the patient.

As a side note, most of this country's doctors, nurses, and medical leaders are caring, compassionate, and skilled people. But they are working in a broken system. David Goldhill, one-time CEO of Game Show Network, lost his father to medical mistakes in a New York hospital, and in 2013, wrote a book about our medical system, entitled *Catastrophic Care: How the American Medical System Killed My Father.* He says it well:

> Accidentally, but relentlessly, America has built a health-care system with incentives that inexorably generate terrible and perverse results. Incentives that emphasize health care over any other aspects of health and well-being. That emphasize treatment over prevention. That disguise true cost. That favor complexity, and discourage transparent competition based on price and quality. That result in a generational pyramid scheme rather than sustainable financing. And that—most importantly—removes consumers from our irreplaceable role as the ultimate insurer of value.

It is my hope that this guide will touch off a movement of skepticism and wisdom in confronting some of life's most difficult choices. If it extends one life or changes one end-of-life course, I will be excited.

PART I

THE MEDICAL ENVIRONMENT IN AMERICA AND YOUR RESPONSE

CHAPTER 1

A BROKEN SYSTEM AND A NATION

GOING BACKWARDS IN LONGEVITY

First, do no harm
—HIPPOCRATES OF KOS

If you really want to understand what's going on in American medicine today, don't just follow the science, follow the money.

The scene is played out tens of thousands of times each year in American hospitals. A patient lies helpless in an intensive care unit, heavily sedated, sometimes restrained, and often intubated so he cannot speak. He is isolated from family members. Meanwhile, his loved ones sit waiting, hoping against hope that technology can give him another shot at life, as sincere critical-care specialists offer shreds of hope and describe flashes of improvement, only to eventually admit defeat.

In August 2012, in Fairfield, Ohio, this scene happened to someone who was no ordinary citizen. Lying in the intensive care unit, clinging to life, was the first man to set foot on the moon, Neil Armstrong. He was a person of faith and a vigorous eighty-two-year-old. A few days earlier, he had walked into his family doctor's office with some moderate heart symptoms. He ended up in the local hospital, where he was advised to undergo coronary bypass surgery. He signed the papers, the surgery was performed, and then a cascade of postoperative procedures and complications left him nonviable even before he went off to the ICU for more than a week.[1] An appalling story, you say, but what does it have to do with the overall care system in this country? To lower his operative risk, perhaps Armstrong should have gone right down the road to Cleveland Clinic, the world pioneer in heart bypass surgery, instead of letting his local hospital talk him into having the procedure done in his hometown?

No, his tragedy was not selecting the wrong hospital to have the surgery performed—it was agreeing to have the surgery performed at all. He made the assumption, based on unsubstantiated advice, that bypass surgery was indicated for his condition and that arduous coronary artery bypass grafting (CABG), would likely extend his life *more than conservative treatment.*[2] As you can see in our footnote and in our heart chapter, that's a dubious and unwise assumption. That's what we mean by overtreatment! Would Cleveland Clinic also have recommended CABG for Armstrong? We'll never know. We do know that this American hero didn't get the medical wisdom he needed.

David S. Jones of Harvard University points out in his book *Broken Hearts: The Tangled History of Cardiac Care* that even though CABG rates in the United States are five to six times higher than in Ontario, Canada, the two have completely comparable heart disease survival rates. Armstrong, who never had a heart attack, made the mistake of assuming that the $75,000 procedure he was being offered was his very best option for an extended life.

Because of his fame, world hero status, and the loyalty of his two sons, Neil Armstrong's family got a $6 million payment from the hospital, in return for no admission of fault and a confidentiality agreement. But that small comfort did not remove his family from the ranks of tens of

thousands of other families who made a series of fateful medical decisions—decisions that seemed wise at the time, but ultimately ended with
premature death or death under agonizing circumstances.

A recent *New York Times* article about the Armstrong family's
tragedy treats Armstrong's death as an unfortunate but somewhat
anomalous event, perhaps rising to the level of substandard care.[3] But
cases like his are not rare anomalies. Armstrong's fate and other celebrity
cases that make it to the popular press—like comedienne Joan Rivers's
throat endoscopy that went very wrong,[4] Andy Warhol's gallbladder
removal that turned tragic through a horrifying mistake in post-op care
in 1987,[5] and comedian Dana Carvey's cardiac bypass in 1998, in which
the wrong artery was bypassed, show us that anyone can be a victim.
They are symbols of a pervasive problem that has overtaken American
medicine. In the context of huge growth in complicated procedures
and increased use of multiple interacting drugs, medical mistakes have
become the third leading cause of death in the United States.

That startling assertion has moved past marginalized circles and
into the mainstream literature of medicine. And it means that you and
I need to shift our approach to medical care or risk being part of this
national tragedy. It has become a life-or-death matter for us.

In 2000, an organization called Institute of Medicine (IOM) released
a study of patient harm called "To Err Is Human: Building a Safer Health
System." It posited up to 98,000 preventable deaths per year in hospitals.
The report created a few press ripples and then faded away. The break-
through into mainstream medical reporting has come through the impas-
sioned efforts of Dr. Martin Makary of Johns Hopkins University School
of Medicine. His study was published in one of the "big five" medical
journals, the *British Medical Journal,* in May of 2016.[6] It estimated that
annually more than 250,000 hospital deaths in the US alone are caused
by medical errors, far ahead of car crashes and every other cause of death
except heart disease and cancer. It wasn't easy for Dr. Makary to assemble
statistics for this landmark conclusion when the previous information had
been mostly anecdotal. And here's why.

The Johns Hopkins team explains that the Centers for Disease Control and Prevention's (CDC) way of collecting national health statistics fails to classify medical errors separately on death certificates. The researchers at Johns Hopkins are advocating for updated criteria in true cause of death on death certificates. "Incidence rates for deaths directly attributable to medical care gone awry haven't been recognized in any standardized method for collecting national statistics," writes Makary. He goes on to explain that the international classifications adopted in 1949 did not include any recognition for iatrogenic (physician-caused) disease because it was not recognized as a problem at the time. According to the CDC in 2013, more than 611,000 people died of heart disease, 584,000 died of cancer, and 149,000 died of chronic respiratory disease—the top three causes of death.

But this newly calculated figure for medical errors in hospitals alone would move this cause of death to number three according to Makary— behind heart disease and cancer, but ahead of respiratory disease. The rank of a cause of death as reported by the CDC is the basis for funding priorities. Since medical mistakes don't appear on the list, it is understandable that very few resources have been allocated to solving them.

After Makary's work brought medical errors into the mainstream, CNBC reporter Ray Sipherd did a commendable follow-up in February of 2018 pointing out that appeals to the CDC to change the way it collects data from death certificates have not been answered.[7] To the date of this writing, no changes have been made.

The CNBC report also points out that the 250,000 deaths include only hospital-related deaths, so it substantially underestimated the issue by any measure, perhaps by an order of magnitude. This had already been recognized by the *Journal of Patient Safety*.[8] In 2013, the *Journal* put the inpatient and outpatient total of preventable deaths in the US at more than 400,000 per year.

And then medical columnist Dr. Gary Kohls points out that even these numbers do not take into account the 50,000 opioid overdose deaths annually, many of which were prescribed by health care providers.

Nor do the numbers account for the thousands of suicides associated with psychiatric drugs, the thousands of heart attacks from NSAIDs, or the thousands of premature deaths from chemotherapy, which are currently included in the cancer death category. Says Dr. Kohls, "One also wonders that if accurate figures were available, combining inpatient and outpatient iatrogenic deaths together (a rational approach) it would cause heart and cancer deaths to drop to number 2 and number 3."[9]

Joe and Teresa Graedon, bestselling authors of *The People's Pharmacy*, came up with the highest annual iatrogenic death total of all, an astounding 788,558—all footnoted with full citations in their newest book.[10] That number, if believable, would catapult medical mistakes and unnecessary deaths to first place, ahead of heart disease in the US. That number would not make the medical establishment happy, but it would indicate the profession's need to get a handle on this problem.

Not only do many of us die early, but many of us "die badly." Dr. Ira Byock, director of a Robert Wood Johnson program on end-of-life care, also leads a team that treats and counsels patients with advanced illnesses.[11] He says modern medicine has become so good at keeping the terminally ill alive at tremendous expense by treating the complications of underlying disease that the inevitable process of dying has become much harder and is often prolonged unnecessarily.

An overwhelming number of people—93% in one study—say they want to die at home surrounded by people they love.[12] Only 25% get to do that. Seventy-five percent of Americans die in a hospital. An astounding 18 to 20% die in an ICU, isolated from everyone they know.[13] And this was before the coronavirus pandemic and the national rush to create thousands of ICU beds and manufacture hundreds of thousands of excess ventilators.

"Families cannot imagine there could be anything worse than their loved one dying. But in fact, there are things much worse. Most generally, it's having someone you love, die badly," Byock says.

A NATION GOING BACKWARDS

All of this has taken a toll on the position of the US in terms of world health indicators, based on longevity. Of course, America is a much larger and more diverse society than some countries it is compared to. But of thirteen countries in a recent comparison, the US ranks twelfth for sixteen available health indicators, including longevity.[14] In another study, the US ranks fifteenth amongst twenty-five industrialized countries on some of the same health indicators.[15]

This is often explained away by saying that the American public engages in bad behaviors: smoking, drinking, drug use, poor eating habits, and perpetrating violence. That's clearly always been a factor in America. But those issues turn out to be a stable factor, not an increasing one. Another factor often cited in American health concerns is income inequality and limited access to health care. That is an alarming social injustice that must be corrected on a high-priority basis. But access to health care among the poor has actually improved marginally over recent years, studies say. For instance, in 2010, 37 million people were uninsured in America; by 2018 that number had shrunk to 23 million.[16] Increasingly, it is recognized that neither of these causes is the driver in declining longevity. David Goldhill states, "Increasingly, researchers are being driven to the recognition of the harmful effects of health care interventions and the likely possibility that they account for a substantial proportion of the excess deaths in the US compared with other comparably industrialized nations."[17]

All these excess and premature deaths show up in individual disease categories because they don't have their own category, making data collection on this topic difficult but not impossible. The data is hiding in plain sight. But you have to know where to look.

For most leading causes of death, mortality rates are higher in the US than in comparable countries. That includes infant mortality and maternal mortality. And then, to add insult to injury, other wealthy countries spend about half as much per person on health care as the US spends.

In the next chapter, we will lay out the principles that enable us to confront proposed treatments with wisdom and discernment. And the following chapters will explore the epidemic of unnecessary diagnostics, drugs, treatments, and devices that most often lead to cascades of adverse events. The purpose of this guide is to prevent heartache and regret and to allow wise and discerning people to live lives uninterrupted by the third leading cause of death in the US, iatrogenic disease. We leave the reformation of the runaway American medical system to others. Our goal is simpler: to protect the lives of those who want to pursue medical wisdom.

—FURTHER READING—

Robert Pearl, MD, *Why We Think We're Getting Good Healthcare and Why We're Usually Wrong* (Philadelphia: Perseus Books, 2017).

Dr. Pearl's book is the most recent of the potential blockbusters that have somehow failed to start a reformation movement even though they have the potential to do so. Dr. Pearl is a caring reconstructive surgeon who was CEO of Kaiser Permanente Medical Group, one of the nation's largest health care providers. He is on the faculty at both Stanford Medical School and Stanford Business School. He went through the untimely death of his father, which occasioned the book. Dr. Pearl's book has been endorsed by bestselling physician-author Atul Gawande. The facts in the book and the credentials of the author have all the makings of a reformation movement. The lack of popular press attention and the peer silence demonstrate just how entrenched this problem is.

CHAPTER 2

THE BASIS FOR MEDICAL WISDOM

AND THE SEVEN KEY QUESTIONS

A friend said to me recently, "I have a legal officer on my team at work, an HR person, and a CFO. I second-guess them all. I even push back on my broker, who has been in the business for thirty years—and once in a while I'm right. But I pretty much do as my doctor says—there's something about that white coat and knowing he's got a whole separate vocabulary he has to dumb down for me. I'm not comfortable engaging that much with him."

Today there are many more reasons to hold that traditional view of your doctor's advice. Medical knowledge is galloping forward at warp speed. Misinformation is rampant on the Internet. The average patient walks in having already looked up his complaint, making the doctor's job harder. Chances are your primary care doctor has invested many hours in staying current, in addition to all the burdensome new office practice requirements laid on him or her and the tremendous pressures of the pandemic in 2020.

And there are many reasons to admire the dedication and motives of primary care doctors. They have chosen to be on the front lines of medicine, even though they could be much more highly compensated as specialists.[1] They are losing the freedom to practice as they see fit, having to consider the desires of third parties such as managed care, lawyers, and their employers. They have to consider the possibility of future lawsuits when making medical decisions, which generally leads to erring on the side of running more tests, recommending more screenings, prescribing more drugs, and offering more procedures. And while taking an aggressive approach often provides the most legal protection for practitioners, health insurance companies make their money, in part, by denying claims—so many physicians find themselves spending additional hours each week arguing for insurance companies to cover the care that they have recommended.

Complicating things further, federal mandates often force doctors to spend more time looking at electronic health records than at their patients. After many previous decades of historic job satisfaction and reward for their hard work, they find their compensation declining as their cost of education increases. As telehealth and urgent care facilities depersonalize medicine even more, and as primary care doctors and even some specialists find themselves being replaced by physician assistants and nurse practitioners, physicians by the thousands are looking for alternatives like concierge medicine—or leaving medicine altogether.

And yet, in light of the facts in the preceding chapter and all the harms that befall ordinary patients in the medical system today, it's urgent that we form partnerships with our primary care doctors to protect ourselves from unwise decisions. I'm an optimist. I believe thoughtful primary care doctors will actually prefer wise patients who have assumed primary responsibility for their own health and are in the office to discuss what's best for them in the long run.

So now that you understand the alarming trends in American medicine (chapter 1) and want to be among that fortunate minority of people who will not follow the crowd—who will use the medical system well and avoid harm—how do you actually learn to be medically wise?

I've created a few steps to follow here and some questions the medically wise person can use to discern wise medical advice from potentially harmful advice.

Armed with these tools, in the following chapters we can look at the most common ways patients get drawn into medical harm today and learn just enough about each specialty to apply our questions intelligently.

The first step in being medically wise is to aspire to it. To recognize that while wisdom always operates with knowledge, wisdom is more than knowledge. It has an intuitive side—and an experience-based side. And for people of faith, there's a spiritual connection; wisdom often comes from outside of us. In the Old Testament, when Solomon asked for wisdom, God was pleased and gave it to him (2 Chronicles 1:11-12). In the New Testament, James enjoins us to ask for wisdom (James 1:5). And Solomon says, in beautiful language, that one of the blessings of wisdom is a tendency toward a long life (Proverbs 3:16). There is never a guarantee, of course, but wisdom in a medical context does increase the odds of living a full life.

The second step in becoming medically wise is to recognize that you are in charge of your health, and it's unwise to cede that responsibility to anyone else—even someone else with superior knowledge. Your doctor's superior knowledge does not trump other pressures he or she is under—for instance, to enforce the practice's so-called standard of care. Again, for people of faith, the Christian Scriptures do not support subrogation of that responsibility to anyone else (I Corinthians 6:19). So even though it is scary, we need to go into every medical encounter with the quiet assurance that we are in charge—legally, morally, and by Scriptural command. Dr. Nortin Hadler of UNC-Chapel Hill Medical

School, one of the favorite authors I quote in this guide, reminds us that the aggressive medical climate today requires wisdom. "You will not be well served," he says, "by bringing either *trust* or *naivete* with you to today's encounters."

The third step to facilitate being medically wise is to create a partnership with your primary care doctor, if you can. This may seem like a daunting task, but a doctor who understands you and your goal of wisdom and conservative medicine is an invaluable asset.

The approach to every doctor will be different and, honestly, won't be successful in every case. But one way to start is to tell doctors you know about the pressure they are under to provide you with a high standard of care, but you'd like them to consider joining forces with you to provide more conservative, carefully considered care. Tell them you're aware that although many people are on multiple medications by the time they are your age, that's not true in Europe and you want to be more conservative. Ask them if they are willing to take the time to give you all the options in a medical situation, from watchful waiting to immediate high-tech treatment. Ask if they would be willing to read and critique this book. Ask if they would sometimes be willing to consider taking a more cautious approach in a situation where their practice's standard of care called for aggressive treatment.

I think you'll find a lot of quiet sympathy out there on the questions of the overdiagnosis and overtreatment that dominates today's medical practice. But as a practical matter, not all physicians feel able to help you be wise. Some just want you to be compliant, as the terminology goes. The larger the organization the doctor works for, the more reluctant he or she may be to form a relationship and help you be medically wise. The physicians' employer has set productivity standards for them, often fifteen minutes per patient, including assistant time, and they may feel under the gun.

What to do then? You may just need to deal with your doctor item by item. An example of that kind of conversation is Appendix 1 in the back of this guide. As a backup, you can get very good at this style of conversation.

The last alternative is to change doctors, if that is practical. An independent practitioner is always a good prospect. But the primary goal is to inspire your current doctor to work with you as you respectfully advance the simple goal of medical wisdom, leading to a long life free of medical harm.

THE POWER OF QUESTIONS

Now we come to the heart of our book. You aspire to wisdom, you're willing to take charge of your medical fate, and you are ready to forge a partnership with your doctor. But what tools do you use? The answer is powerful clarifying questions—among the most useful things in any area of life. My terrific CEO coach for many years, Bobb Biehl, is a master at the art of the powerful question. From him, I learned that *when all the facts are in, the answers jump out at you.* And in medicine, the way you get all the facts in and let real science triumph is through insightful questions that hopefully pierce through false assumptions, biases, third-party influences, and massaged data. So here are the questions. Let's be clear about our powerful questions, though. Answering "yes" to any of these questions *does not* mean you should decline the services being offered. It *does* alert you to the fact that the decision requires further investigation—it moves proposals of medications or procedures from the "easy" category to the "medical wisdom required" category, where you keep gaining knowledge until the answer jumps out at you.

1. *Is the primary goal of this medication or procedure to relieve a symptom? Do we know anything about the underlying cause of this symptom?*
Symptomatic treatment, if clearly and honestly defined and labeled, is today's dominant modality. It comprises most of the drugs advertised on TV, though the advertisers might vigorously debate that. A *yes* to this question should always trigger further fact finding. Treating symptoms, not causes, is an issue that needs to be honestly confronted by every medically wise patient who presents a serious symptom to his or

her doctor. We all know that when we take an over-the-counter pain reliever, we're not doing anything about the original source of the pain, and deep down we know we should stop to consider the source. But we often don't because the stakes don't seem high.

But when you consider taking a new drug to relieve the symptoms of a serious autoimmune disease such as Crohn's disease, the stakes are a lot higher. There are no drugs available that address the poorly understood underlying causes of this autoimmune disease. That's right: no matter how high-tech they sound, the only widely available class of drug you can take today is one that suppresses the symptoms of Crohn's by suppressing targeted parts of your immune system. That fact is certainly not promoted on TV or even stated to patients today, unless you are medically wise enough to ask. But this is not a diatribe against a drug like Humira. If I had the very distressing symptoms of Crohn's disease, I might well take Humira. This is a call to see whether you are treating symptoms not the disease; if you take an immunosuppressant long enough, serious things can and probably will happen to you.

Any medically wise person should first ask this question—am I treating symptoms when I have a chance to address the underlying condition? Sometimes the answer is that I have no insight into reversing the condition through diet, through stress reduction, through alternative medicine and the like. But the wise person always asks the question. In gallbladder disease, for instance, there *are* alternatives to simply removing the organ, which sometimes amounts to symptomatic treatment. We hope you recognize plenty of examples in succeeding chapters for applying this question.

2. *Is this a recommendation for treatment of indefinite length?*
This second question is the one that can tip you off to look into your medical future. If you are prescribed a drug with no ending date to prevent a condition or control a symptom, then you have moved from the ranks of well person to permanent patient. This has been normalized in American medicine, although not so much in Europe. There's

no larger factor associated with today's overdiagnosis and overtreatment epidemic than this statistic—almost 70% of American adults are on at least one medication long term.[2] Today, we think that's normal. But the life insurance companies are not fooled when compiling their actuarial tables. They reduce your life expectancy, as they should. I realize it all sounds so logical, and lab tests don't lie, but we all need to consider the long-term consequences of not addressing the underlying cause in any meaningful way and of taking symptom-relieving medications indefinitely. Long-term drug use has consequences. Chapters 3 and 4 address this question in detail. The bottom line is that medications with "forever refills" may be better for the drug companies than for you.

3. *Is this condition causing me symptoms or was it diagnosed solely through lab results?*

Let's first say that laboratory tests can be very valuable. Many developing conditions are first revealed in lab tests. Liver enzyme abnormalities can signal developing liver disease before you feel anything, for instance. Pap smears can detect incipient cervical cancer long before women sense anything is wrong.

At the same time, laboratory results today enable overdiagnosis. The threshold of many "popular diseases" is being defined down, and lab results are leading to treatments that don't show positive risk/benefit ratios. They are putting millions of people on permanent prescriptions with inferred and unverified benefits. Do you have "high blood pressure"? Well now the definition of "elevated blood pressure" is anything above 120 systolic. It used to be 140. You'll find this topic treated in chapters 2 and 3.

Do you have type 2 diabetes? You are many times more likely to be told that you do than in 1990. The definitions have gotten much tighter. Isn't this good, you say? We're catching things much earlier. That makes a good story, but you'll see in later chapters that lifestyle changes to counter incipient diabetes are a much better bet. Early diagnosis is certainly good for the pharmaceutical companies, but a lifetime of chasing A1C while taking high-tech drugs is not medical wisdom. The science just isn't there on the benefits of long-term medication for people with "marginally abnormal" lab results.

So lab results with no symptoms mean one of two things—they are valuable early warnings of disease, or they are unwise ways to make you a permanent patient. It is your job as a medically wise person to discern which.

4. *Is this finding related to the reason for which I saw my doctor or had this test—or is it a completely incidental finding?*

Here we have another question that presumes you are asymptomatic— you feel well. Or perhaps you are being treated for another condition, and a scan that reaches into another body area shows a potentially scary situation for which you are totally unprepared. Could it be something serious? Should you let your doctor trigger a full investigation?

Millions of *incidentalomas*, medical slang for unrelated findings, are found each year. Some people end up very grateful that something was found early and treated successfully. But some people, unwilling to take a chance that it's nothing or told it can't be determined definitively, won't wait and see. They end up being treated very aggressively for something that would have never caused problems.

You say no, that can't happen in the era of high-tech medicine? Oh, yes it can—it happened to a colleague who went through chemotherapy for pancreatic cancer and then a debilitating Whipple procedure for an incidentaloma—which turned out to be scary but benign. A yes to our fourth question should put your medical wisdom antennae up in full alert mode, ready to follow the science to the very end rather than opting for opinions early. This question is highly relevant in chapters 5, 6, 7, and 8. (By the way, most incidentalomas turn out to not be life threatening.)

5. *Is the fear factor getting in the way of my rational decision-making process?*

When we use the word *fear* in a medical context, the first thing that comes to mind is cancer, so chapter 7 is going to be your best teacher. The key to this question is making decisions on a rational, scientific, and medical-wisdom basis even when you're afraid. Courage is not the absence of fear, of course; it's doing the right thing in the presence of fear. So how do you step outside of your own emotions to trust in God and make wise decisions in a serious situation?

One way is to practice for big life events, just as pilots do for all sorts of aviation emergencies in flight simulators or in the air. My own pilot training has helped me here. If I were given a life-threatening diagnosis, what are the first, second, and third things I would do? There's a cancer-related list in chapter 7. Another way is to make friends and allies whom you know to be medically wise. There aren't many candidates with that kind of wisdom, but friends who have a kind of settled wisdom are like gold when fear intervenes.

6. *Has my personal risk of disease or an adverse event been explained to me in terms of <u>relative risk</u> or <u>absolute risk</u>?*

This question requires the most reasoning power of any of our seven questions. You might be saying, "I'm not a scientist, a math major, or even a person with any interest in statistics." But bear with me for a few moments. Let's understand how statistics are being used today in medicine and take another step toward being a medically wise person.

Relative risk is the single most useful tool in the toolbox for drug marketers today and the basis for setting recommendations and protocols for various diagnoses, procedures, and even surgeries. This specialized kind of statistical thinking has even polluted the "big five" peer-reviewed medical journals today, and editors have resigned over it. But what is the difference between relative risk and absolute risk, you say?

Here's an example from John Abramson, MD, on the subject of osteoporosis in mature women and a randomized clinical trial on a drug called Fosamax, published in *Journal of the American Medical Association* (*JAMA*), way back in 1998. In that study, it was claimed that the women (with an average age of sixty-eight) who took Fosamax for four years were 56% less likely to suffer a hip fracture than the women in a control group. Impressive? Now, let's let Dr. Abramson translate that into absolute risk:

> This sounds like very good news for women with osteoporosis, but how many hip fractures were really prevented? With no drug therapy at all, women with osteoporosis had a 99.5% chance of making it through each year without a hip fracture—pretty good odds. With drug therapy, their odds improved to 99.8%. In other words, taking the drugs decreased their risk of hip fracture from 0.5% per year to 0.2% per year. This tiny decrease in absolute risk translates into the study's reported 56% reduction in relative risk. The bottom line is that 81 women with osteoporosis have to take Fosamax for 4.2 years at a cost of more than $300,000 to prevent one hip fracture.[3]

In succeeding chapters, we will give other examples of relative risk used to market drugs—drugs which presumably would have fewer sales if people understood their medical situation in terms of real risk rather than relative risk. Another prime example is atrial fibrillation and the so-called blood thinners so heavily advertised today. A-fib is now a household word and has become a burgeoning medical industry based on relative risk numbers, so it's worth understanding a little bit about statistics in order to be medically wise.

7. *Do I feel pressure to make a significant medical decision on the spot?*

There are times in life when emergencies demand an on-the-spot decision. You pray, bring all your life experience to bear, and make a decision for yourself or your loved one right then. But most medical decisions are not like that. Most medication and procedure decisions are elective—as the medical profession likes to say. And in that context, if you feel pressured, making a decision right then is *always* a bad idea. In fact, it's a much worse idea than doing the same thing at a car dealership. There's a lot more to lose. And sometimes the pressure can be artificial, not appropriate to the real context. Examples of pressure-filled situations are the stuff of hospital medical dramas on television, but most often not in real life.

At the risk of being very prescriptive here, I'll tell you what I think constitutes medical wisdom in the face of decision pressure. Make major medical decisions only after an independent consultation. Friends of your doctor in the same practice group or online sources run by the big hospital groups sadly do not constitute an independent second opinion in my view. They don't always present a fresh perspective—they end up as variants on the same line of reasoning.

Independent second opinions are the ones you find from your own research or networking. In the preface to this guide, I tell the story of a second opinion from a cardiologist I networked with. She gave me a whole new view of the meaning of my stress test, EKG, and echocardiogram done by an interventional cardiologist a few weeks before. It defused pressure and was hugely liberating. I am still grateful.

There may well be other wisdom-based questions I've missed that could show up in the second edition of this guide. But as you move on to specific areas of medical knowledge that you need to learn about, let's apply these seven questions. I believe they are the foundation of your path to wisdom and a life lived clear of the overdiagnosis and overtreatment epidemic we have in American medicine today.

PART II

THE KEY DANGERS FOR YOU

CHAPTER 3

GET OVERDIAGNOSED AND

BECOME A PERMANENT PATIENT

Allowing yourself to get caught in and harmed by today's broken American health system is relatively easy: *simply let yourself be diagnosed with something that has never caused you symptoms and will never lead to your death.* You will not be alone. Americans today are overdiagnosed by the millions. Then they are treated, mostly with drugs, but also with procedures. Many experience harm. All experience the subtle psychological change that moves them from *well person* to *patient.*

Dr. Gil Welch, a renowned authority on the effects of medical screening and former head of Dartmouth's Institute for Health Policy and Clinical Practice, defines overdiagnosis this way: "Over-diagnosis is when individuals are identified, labeled, and treated for conditions that will never cause symptoms or death."[1] That's worth a few moments of meditation.

A NATION OF PATIENTS

By the time they are fifty, most Americans are on prophylactic or symptom-suppressing medications—typically antihypertensives for blood pressure, statins for "hyperlipidemia" (see chapter 8), medications for prediabetic high blood sugar, or much worse, blood thinners for atrial fibrillation, or immunosuppressants for GI conditions, skin conditions or arthritis. As we said, 60% of American adults now live with the diagnosis of at least one chronic condition.[2]

A NEW PHENOMENON

This wasn't true a couple of generations ago. One reason is that the standards for defining all these diseases have been tightened year after year in the name of prevention. But as that happens, more people can become permanent patients and revenue generators. The goal posts for being diseased have been moved without our knowledge or consent, or more importantly, our primary care provider's consent.

On the diabetes front, for instance, the definition of a type 2 diabetic used to be a fasting blood sugar over 140 mg/dl. Now it's 126 mg/dl, turning 1.6 million people into permanent "diabetes patients."[3]

Isn't this good, you ask? Aren't we preventing bigger problems later on? Certainly, in the case of extremely high blood sugar, the risk/benefit ratio makes medicating appropriate. But in mild cases, it is much less clear. Statistically speaking, the number of people you need to treat to prevent one person from getting worse is often in the hundreds. More on that later. Then, there is the fact that each of these prophylactic treatments has a possible long-term downside even beyond its short-term side effects. That's our next chapter.

As the threshold for diagnosing many common conditions comes down, there are four societal effects: 1) millions more people become permanent patients, 2) billions of dollars pour into the coffers of pharmaceutical companies, 3) thousands of patients suffer side effects for every person helped, and 4) many people are harmed or have their lives shortened for reasons we will explore throughout this book. Iatrogenic disease expert Dr. Gil Welch illustrates why medicating borderline patients is not always good:

> This is not a happy story. Mr. Roberts was a seventy-four-year old man whose major medical problem was ulcerative colitis, but well managed. One day, in a routine lab test, Mr. Roberts was found to have elevated blood sugar. It wasn't that high, but the finding prompted more testing. And more testing confirmed the diagnosis: diabetes. He had type 2 diabetes. ... Although he had no symptoms of diabetes, over the past few decades, doctors had gotten much more aggressive about treating it early, so his primary care physician started him on glyburide—a drug that lowers blood sugar. The medication worked well.
>
> Six months later he blacked out while driving on the local interstate. His car went off the road and rolled over. ... The medication had worked too well. I'd hate to have been the doctor who prescribed him glyburide.
>
> But I was that doctor. Mr. Roberts was in the hospital for over a month. ... I felt terrible. It goes without saying—I didn't restart the glyburide. Mr. Roberts is now ninety and still a patient of mine. He has not been treated for diabetes since the accident, nor has he had any complications from diabetes. I think he was over-diagnosed. But he was lucky. There was no permanent injury.

THE BLOOD PRESSURE OVERTREATMENT EPIDEMIC

The same thing is happening with what is now called *elevated blood pressure*. It's clear that out-of-control blood pressure, let's say 200 systolic/115 diastolic, can lead to strokes, heart failure, kidney damage, and eye hemorrhage. But today, elevated blood pressure is defined as anything over 120/80. In their defense, most physicians wait to see a rising pattern, take the pressure multiple times, and employ other cautions before prescribing. But the new protocols are staring them in the face and making them less conservative.

In the appendix to this guide, I create an imaginary conversation between a doctor and a patient to illustrate an adept patient who escapes overtreatment for elevated blood pressure while maintaining the relationship.

UNDERSTANDING THE RISK/BENEFIT

There is a concept in medical research called "number needed to treat." For example, you need to treat nineteen patients with borderline hypertension to reduce the chance of an event like a stroke happening in one patient. So if you are diagnosed with borderline hypertension and get on medication, you can be one of the lucky 6% who actually benefit in some way. The rest, 94%, will not benefit.[4] And the market for prehypertension is even larger than for prediabetes, some eighteen million Americans.[5] You are on the medication for years—as long as your physician can persuade you to take it.

Meanwhile, the longer you take these medications, which are usually diuretics, various ACE inhibitors, calcium channel blockers, or beta blockers, the more you are exposed to their long-term effects. Some diuretics, for instance, make it harder for your body to maintain potassium balance, putting stress on your heart. ACE inhibitors interfere with your body's ability to constrict blood vessels. Beta and calcium blockers can prevent your heart from responding to increased demands for blood by beating faster. None of these classes of drugs address the underlying blood pressure problem, whatever that may be. All of those side effects may be worth it in cases of severe hypertension, but in cases of borderline hypertension, it is unclear if the risks of these drugs outweigh the benefits.

Here's what to do about this if you are diagnosed with borderline hypertension: work with your doctor to understand what class of hypertension you fall into and the class of drug you will receive. Ask for any benefit studies that might exist in your class with the suggested treatment. Study the numbers if any can be provided. Ask about lifestyle changes you can make first. Read the imaginary conversation in the back of this guide. Then make your own informed decision.

HIGHER RISK OVERDIAGNOSIS

The stakes are much higher if your doctor or a specialist advises you to go on the so-called blood thinners (anticoagulants) or immunosuppressant drugs. You and your doctor may decide that these are necessary to remove a clear and present danger to your life on a short- or medium-term basis. But today these drugs are marketed heavily on television for long-term users. From all I have read, few patients escape without complications. You have become among the most unfortunate of permanent patients, living on borrowed time, waiting for the next complication. Let's look at each of these drug classes one at a time, starting with blood thinners. Drugs like Pradaxa, Savaysa, Eliquis, and Xarelto, with new ones coming out all the time, are highly touted as superior to older drugs such as warfarin. Their use can be a reasonable idea for a limited time after surgery. If you have been unfortunate enough to have a stent put in one of your arteries even though you have never had a heart attack (see chapter 8), then they are necessary for a time. Or if you have had a DVT (deep vein thrombosis), it is wise to be on a clot preventer for the limited time your doctor recommends.

But the growth market for these drugs is for another application: to reduce stroke risks in people who have had episodes of an abnormal heart rhythm called atrial fibrillation, sometimes asymptomatic. In the US, over 5.2 million people are estimated to be living with A-fib, as it's often called.[6] Estimates are imprecise, and no one actually knows the prevalence of the condition, although the incidence certainly rises with age. But A-fib is a condition being diagnosed more frequently and rising fast in public consciousness, partially due to large investments in advertising by the makers of anticoagulants like Eliquis. There's a battle for the top spot in the growing blood thinner market, and A-fib is the top application. The reservoir of possible patients seems almost limitless.

But here is the dilemma with A-fib and blood thinners for the medically wise person. It is widely quoted in the advertising for anticoagulants that A-fib increases the risk of a stroke by up to five times above the general population. But this is a classic generalized relative risk statement. We learned about relative risk in chapter 2. Firstly, if you have this condition, your actual risk varies widely depending on many facts—a new "CHADS score" helps cardiologists get to your personal risk.

But secondly, and more importantly, you need to know your absolute risk. As best as you can determine, what is the actual percentage of likelihood that A-fib patients like you will have a stroke this year? And then, if you decide to take one of the new blood thinners to reduce your risk, by how much will it reduce your risk?

And then, what is the absolute risk for a serious or fatal bleeding event on this medication? Is the absolute risk of a bleeding event higher or lower than your risk of a stroke? These are legitimate and important questions for you. The wise patient takes note of the fact that this information is not easily available either to physicians or patients at this writing. The medically wise person tries to get a handle on the facts before starting a blood thinner medication, which is a serious and powerful drug.

IMMUNOSUPPRESSANTS AND YOU

Now, we finally come to the most risk-laden class of commonly prescribed drugs—ones on which to exercise much medical wisdom before taking. These are the heavily advertised immunosuppressants such as Xeljanz, Humira, Cosentyx, Azasan, Arava, Orencia, Enbrel, Remicade, and Rituxan, to name a few. They are marketed for serious autoimmune conditions like lupus, rheumatoid arthritis, Crohn's disease, and multiple sclerosis. They are also being marketed for less serious but distressing conditions such as alopecia and psoriasis.

The marketing is a combination of lawyer-like wording (Humira *may* lower your ability to fight infections) and recitations of dire complications and side effects, repeated so often that TV viewers become inured to them.

Immunosuppressants are not new. Organ transplant patients know they have to live with the threat of these complications for the rest of their lives. What is new is that people like you and me are willing to trade off the risks of a suppressed immune system against the hope that we will be lucky and not have serious complications. These drugs have been certified safe and effective by the FDA, but every physician knows that prescribing certain immunosuppressive drugs puts their patients at an increased risk of serious infections, cancer, and cardiovascular disease. And while the side effects are required to be mentioned, their incidence rate is much harder to find. Try to find data on the incidence of T-cell lymphoma from one of the major immunosuppressants, for instance. It's not easily available, but you can dig for it, and we tackle that in the next chapter. But it's clear that thousands of ordinary people who were prescribed a drug for a bothersome ailment like psoriasis or a more debilitating ailment like Crohn's disease are now fighting for their lives after developing T-cell lymphoma or some other potentially fatal complication. The growth of this class of drug—fueled by "new applications" and direct-to-consumers (DTC) TV advertising—is a compounded 14% per year.[7]

One thing is clear: patients taking immunosuppressants on a long-term basis are more likely to die in any one year as a result of suppressing their immune systems than the general population. We just don't know how much more likely. That information isn't publicly available because the manufacturers have little incentive to do extensive research on long-term effects. Hopefully the information provided in the next chapter will give you reason to look carefully into any drug that suppresses your immune system.

There are many more examples of overdiagnosis and overtreatment through aggressive protocols, such as the tests for osteoporosis and treatment for marginal liver enzyme abnormalities, that this chapter does not have space to treat.

The bottom line is this: if a doctor tells you, as a result of testing, that you need to go on a medication indefinitely (in other words, become a permanent patient), stop the train, get off, and read up on your specific condition, its relative risk to you, and the risk/benefit ratio.

You have to decide what you want your physical life to look like when you are seventy. Unfortunately, you and your doctor can't depend on today's aggressive protocols and profit-driven medications to promote your best interest.

—THE FACTS—

- Sixty percent of all Americans over fifty are now described as having a chronic condition and are on long-term medications. [8]

- Millions are being medicated because of borderline test numbers with unknown risk/benefit ratios, as our chapter has demonstrated.

- This epidemic of overtreatment grows yearly as disease is redefined by guideline makers in conjunction with pharmaceutical influences.

- The most prevalent and egregious overtreatment occurs with cases of borderline high blood sugar, borderline high blood pressure, and alleged high cholesterol.

—THE PATH OF WISDOM—

- Consider not treating your borderline high blood pressure with drugs. Start with lifestyle changes.

- Consider not treating borderline type 2 diabetes without first looking for lifestyle and dietary changes that will help.

- Consider not starting blood thinners for indefinite use. Find a way to address the underlying condition if you can.

- Consider not starting immunosuppressants for indefinite use if you and your doctor can agree on any other alternatives for treatment.

- Set a goal to live the kind of lifestyle that allows you to skip ongoing use of drugs for as long as you can.

CHAPTER 4

TAKING MEDICATIONS INDEFINITELY WITHOUT KNOWLEDGE OF THEIR LONG-TERM EFFECTS

As we began to illustrate in chapter 3, an important way to become a permanent patient and perhaps shorten your lifespan is to be talked into taking a drug indefinitely without understanding its potential to cause serious long-term effects.

Americans, with 5% of the world's population, take 38% of the world's prescription medicines. Europeans don't take medications at the rate Americans do, partly because they don't get exposed to the hundreds of millions of dollars of direct-to-consumer drug advertising that Americans do. New Zealand is the only other developed country that allows direct-to-consumer marketing of prescription drugs.

So here's the concern, touched on in the preceding chapter but unfolded in detail here: the long-term use of almost any medication is problematic, according to almost anyone except the manufacturer. In some cases, it is even likely to shorten your life—especially if the medication is only controlling the symptoms of a condition, not addressing its cause, as most are.

Many people are vaguely uneasy about the drugs they take but are not sure what to do about it. I encounter this repeatedly.

The setting was beautiful, a garden-like backyard lunch on an early fall afternoon for my wife and me. The other couple learned I was writing a guide for personal protection against medical errors. They were both on Lipitor (atorvastatin), the second most prescribed drug in the US, with 105 million prescriptions written in 2019. It was clear that they were uneasy about its long-term use but had no source for estimating their risk of long-term health-damaging effects. Nor did I at that time. How could this be? There were no clinical studies of the long-term effects of the number two drug in the world, taken by tens of millions of Americans?

It turns out there are some *medium-term* studies on Lipitor, but they are only discoverable by digging through peer-reviewed journals. They get a mention on *WebMD* but only with a phrase. I did some digging. To their credit, independent researchers are looking at the association between the long-term use of Lipitor (atorvastatin) and its rival cousins, pravastatin and rosuvastatin, with respect to the onset of type 2 diabetes.

And here's what a recent journal report said.[1] "More recent meta-analysis of observational trials confirms and reinforces the increased risk of diabetes mellitus with statin use. Although it has been suggested that treatment of 10,000 patients for 5 years with an effective regime (40 mg atorvastatin daily) would yield between 50 and 100 new cases of new-onset type 2 diabetes mellitus, this is far outweighed by the beneficial effects of statins on coronary vessel disease."[2] By the way, that last comment is not only unproven but gratuitous—editorial comments like that have no place in a research article without citations.

In other words, to get all these alleged, unproven cardiovascular benefits, small numbers of patients have to "take one for the team" in terms of acquiring type 2 diabetes. This approach to the long-term effects of popular drugs is not an issue if patients get to understand the risks themselves and then choose the drugs anyway. It is a *big* problem if they know nothing about the risks. That's a problem this chapter is designed to help you with.

How did this situation develop in US medicine?

THE DRUG APPROVAL PROCESS

In the US, the Food and Drug Administration (FDA) is the agency in the executive branch that reports to the president through the US Department of Health and Human Services (HHS) and is responsible for regulating pharmaceuticals and medical devices.

The FDA has a "sophisticated and complex system" for ensuring that drugs are "safe and effective," a phrase that has been in use for decades. The review process is based on ensuring those two qualities. The public's level of knowledge about the FDA's process took a large jump forward during the development of COVID-19 vaccines when Operation Warp Speed achieved the approval of a vaccine in under a year, a tribute to the FDA's flexibility under duress. Many people came away very impressed.

But let's take a look at the process of approving a drug in the context of understanding why long-term dangers remain for many drugs. The process begins in the laboratories of drug manufacturers and startups. The pharmaceutical companies have hundreds of investigations going at any one time, focusing on lab work and animal testing. But when they find something of great interest, they submit a formal investigational new drug application to the FDA. That submission, if approved, allows clinical trials to begin on humans in three phases.

Phase I studies on humans are typically done with about twenty to eighty healthy paid volunteers. The focus in Phase I is on toxicity and safety. If Phase I studies show acceptable levels of side effects and no immediate toxicity, then Phase II begins. This time, the focus is on effectiveness, and the volunteers, from a few dozen to 300 or so, usually have a condition the drug is aimed at affecting positively.

At the end of Phase II, a plan is developed for a major clinical trial, usually up to about 3,000 people (but 20,000 to 40,000 with the COVID vaccines). About that time a formal new drug application (NDA) is submitted.

For standard drugs, the FDA is required by law to agree to review it or reject it within sixty days. Then it is required to complete the review process (for 90% of drugs) within ten months. The Phase III data are also reviewed by an independent review board, which became even more important in Operation Warp Speed for the COVID vaccine. For instance, the emergency use authorization (EUA) for the Pfizer COVID-19 vaccine was approved by the review board by a vote of 17 to 4 with one abstention.

There are criticisms of the process to be sure, mostly focusing on the economic incentives which lead big companies to "reshape" data at times and to write off major fines for doing so as the cost of doing business. And some of the critics who have worked in the industry are outraged. In 2013, Peter Gotzsche wrote a book, *Deadly Medicine and Organized Crime: How Big Pharma has Corrupted Healthcare*, penning over 300 meticulously documented pages.

Some now question the whole process of clinical trials undertaken by the FDA and pharmaceutical companies where the two entities get too cozy. For instance, Marcia Angell, former editor of the prestigious *New England Journal of Medicine,* said in 2010 that "it is simply no longer possible to believe much of the clinical research that is published. … I take no pleasure in this conclusion, which I reached slowly and reluctantly over my two decades as an editor."[3]

But our purpose here is not to reform the FDA or tilt against Big Pharma. Our purpose in this guide is to keep you safe from long-term drug damage. We have two points to make. One is that many highly damaging effects of drugs don't come to light in the relatively short-term time frames of drug approvals, however thorough they may be.

And the second point is that when taken long enough, any drug, that

interferes with the natural processes of the body (let's say its natural pro-
duction of cholesterol, for instance, as statins do) may eventually affect
your lifespan in some way. Let's underline that last point because this is a
major principle in acquiring medical wisdom. Most people do not think
that way about drugs, just as most people think, unwisely, about cancer
in a binary way—e.g., if there are abnormal cells anywhere in your body,
they are going to kill you—and then they act accordingly (see chapter 7).

Here are just three examples of our first point—some drugs don't
give up their secrets until they've been out there a few years.

Such is the family of antibiotics called fluoroquinolones, in wide use
since the 1980s for conditions including acute sinusitis, acute bronchitis,
and uncomplicated urinary tract infections. I have personal experience
with quinolones for possible bacterial prostatitis in the 1990s with
medium-term use, which I would never do again. I would especially
never do it again because my actions were exactly what I warn about in
chapter 10—taking a common complaint with an uncertain diagnosis
and throwing a treatment at it. My final diagnosis for that complaint was
prostadynia, medical talk for pain in the prostate area for which we have
absolutely no explanation. We're complex beings. It finally went away.

Let's return to the story of the quinolones, the most recognizable
brand name of which is Cipro (ciprofloxacin). Reports of serious adverse
events began emerging. In 2008, the FDA put a "black box warning" on
the labels of all quinolones, warning of tendinitis and tendon rupture,
especially in older adults, perhaps hoping that would take care of these
newly discovered dangers.

But it was not to be. In 2011, the FDA was forced to add a warning
for all myasthenia gravis patients of possible worsening of their symptoms. In 2013, it added a warning about irreversible peripheral nerve
damage. In August of 2015, it convened an advisory committee, which
decided that fluoroquinolones should no longer be first-line antibiotics
for common infections. But heavy usage went on. The FDA has now
received more than 60,000 complaints about irreparable harm, and tens
of thousands belong to an online support group describing themselves

as "floxed." In 2018, mental health problems were added to the list for fluoroquinolones. All this emerged more than a decade after initial FDA and independent panel approval. Although the FDA requires manufacturers to keep a log of long-term side effects as a condition of the approval process, the situation has to get pretty bad for the FDA to order a product off the market. Subtle long-term effects don't make the news.

There are many more examples of longer-term adverse effects that do not show up in the approval process. Elmiron (pentosan polysulfate sodium) is a drug for a painful bladder condition called interstitial cystitis—a condition that affects several million Americans each year, many of them women. Elmiron has been on the market since the late 1990s and has provided relief for many, helping with the pain from this incurable condition. Before June of 2020, the labels on Elmiron said nothing about a big problem that was brewing in the background and has now triggered multiple lawsuits. The problem is maculopathy, a condition that can lead to blindness and that many doctors may misdiagnose as age-related macular degeneration.

Probably the most recent and best-known example of a drug with a known long-term side effect is Zantac (ranitidine), approved by the FDA in 1986 and thought to be so benign that it was available in both prescription and over-the-counter strengths to treat heartburn. It turns out Zantac has had a cancer-causing contaminant in it for years called nitrosodimethylamine. The drug has been taken off the market, and lawsuits are piling up.

And now the broader class of drugs to which Zantac belongs, called proton pump inhibitors (PPIs), used to treat heartburn and the more serious esophageal reflux syndrome called GERD, is also in trouble. PPIs are a $10 billion drug class in the US that remain very effective for short-term use. Long-term use is another topic, however, because PPIs inhibit the body's ability to make gastric acid, which protects us in multiple ways. So even the over-the-counter versions of PPIs like Prevacid, Nexium, and Prilosec, if taken long-term, are now associated with increased risk of pneumonia, bone fractures from loss of calcium, acceleration of dementia, and C. difficile colitis. All of this suffering incurred trying to alleviate a condition that is strongly influenced by dietary choices and weight, and that some believe has a strong mind-body connection.

Let us return to our prior topic—patients who are unfortunate enough to be part of the very small percentage who acquire type 2 diabetes from statins. Diabetes is a life-shortening condition, but at least it's manageable. This is not so with the complications that arise from newer, more complex drugs today; many of those complications are very difficult to treat.

For that discussion, let's look at one of the highest revenue drugs in the US today, and one of the most heavily promoted. It's called Humira (adalimumab). US sales were $13.7 billion in 2019. Drug maker AbbVie averages an astounding $5,243 in revenue for every prescription sold.[4] At that price, it certainly might be fair to ask about long-term effects of Humira?

And at that price you might guess Humira is prescribed for a rare stage IV cancer. Nope. It is prescribed for moderate to severe rheumatoid arthritis, psoriasis, Crohn's disease, and a few other conditions, all of them increasing in the US population—a hugely successful drug.

How could it be useful for all these conditions? Because it is an immunosuppressant, and those diseases are all autoimmune conditions. Humira is what's called a tumor necrosis fastor (TNF) blocker, which blocks the activity of TNF, a protein involved in inflammation.

As stated daily on television, side effects of Humira may include tuberculosis; serious viral, bacterial, or fungal infections; and T-cell lymphoma. Doctors generally inform patients of these risks, which increase with long-term use. Fair enough.

But what are the actual plain language risk numbers so that patients can make their own informed decisions? They are researchable, and they are generally available to physicians if they study the prescriptive literature with calculator in hand. But they are not available for consumers in understandable terms. It turns out, for instance, in the clinical trials, that "T-cell lymphoma of a particularly virulent kind has occurred in 3.19 people per 100 patient-years with Humira."[5]

The sample size was 7,800 people. Solving for that, which few physicians would do, means that just .03 patients would get lymphoma per patient year. But multiplying that by a million Humira patients in the last ten years means over 300 unfortunate souls have gotten lymphoma from taking Humira. Again, this poses no problem in the case of truly informed consent for short-term use, but a big problem for long-term use without specific risk numbers.

Humira provides blessed, if sometimes temporary, relief for many sufferers whose lives are miserable. So, many would have elected to try Humira anyway. But the lack of decipherable consumer information for medium-range side effects with Humira, a drug that is doing about $20 billion in world-wide sales per year, needs addressing. If you are taking a long-term drug, you owe it to yourself to know whether it addresses the cause of your condition instead of the symptoms only and know what the long-term risks are. This chapter is hopefully helping with that.

I can tell you on the basis of extensive research that few independent resources are available that can help an ordinary intelligent citizen evaluate the risks from long-term prescription drug use.

Dr. Sidney Wolfe, founder of Public Citizen's Health Research Group, is an exception. He has been on this issue since 1971. He is a pioneer and a hero, and his website at worstpills.org is a source of valuable information on the latest in drug interactions, FDA recalled drugs, and potential short-term risks. But even he does not focus on long-term risks of the most popular classes of drugs or their ability to shorten your lifespan.

So, we have appended to this chapter a sample list of some prescription drugs currently being promoted for long-term use, the conditions they are prescribed for, and references to research going on about their long-term adverse effects. It is far from an exhaustive list—we simply highlight here some drugs for which adverse long-term effects are emerging, to reinforce our point that elective use of long-term drugs may not be wise. I hope each of you are able to live out a full natural life, free from long-term drug-induced chronic conditions.

Generic Name(s)	Brand Name(s)	Condition(s) Treated	Emerging Long-Term Concerns
Adalimumab	Humira	Rheumatoid arthritis Crohn's disease Psoriasis Other autoimmune	Serious infections[6] Heart failure[6] T-cell lymphoma[7]
Beta-blockers Atenolol Metoprolol Propranolol	Lopressor Tenormin Toprol Inderal Hemangeol	Hypertension Angina Atrial fibrillation Tremors	Altered glycemic metabolism[8] Acute delirium[9]
Chlorthalidone	Hygroton Thalitone	Hypertension Edema	Chronic kidney disease[10] Kidney failure[10] Type 2 diabetes[10]
Clopidogrel	Plavix	Deep vein thrombosis Atrial fibrillation Post heart attack Post stent	No further benefit seen after one year[11]
Fluoroquinolones Ciprofloxacin Levofloxacin	Cipro Levaquin	Bacterial infections	Tendon rupture[12] Permanent peripheral neuropathy[13] Liver injury[14]

Generic Name(s)	Brand Name(s)	Condition(s) Treated	Emerging Long-Term Concerns
Furosemide	Lasix	Edema Hypertension Hypercalcemia	Progression of heart failure[15] Increased risk of hospitalization[15] Increased risk of hospitalization[15]
Lisinopril	Lestril Obelis Prinivil	Hypertension	Autoimmune skin blistering[16]
Metformin	Fortamet Glucophage Glumetza Riomet	Type 2 diabetes	Anemia[17]
Pentosan	Elmiron	Interstitial cystitis	Maculopathy leading to blindness[18]
Proton-pump inhibitors Esomeprazole Lansoprazole Omeprazole Pantoprazole	Nexium Prevacid Prilosec Protonix	GERD (heartburn)	Hypergastrin-emia[19] Pneumonia[20] Dementia[21]
Ranitidine	Zantac	GERD (heartburn)	Carcinogen contamination[22]

Generic Name(s)	Brand Name(s)	Condition(s) Treated	Emerging Long-Term Concerns
Rituximab	Rituxan	Autoimmune diseases Some cancers	Difficult-to-treat chronic hepatitis E[23] Increased risk of hospitalization[15]
Statins Atorvastatin Pravastatin Rosuvastatin Simvastatin	Lipitor Pravachol Crestor Zocor	High cholesterol	New onset type 2 diabetes[24] New onset osteoporosis[25] Interstitial lung disease[26] Kidney toxicity[27] Liver toxicity[28] Cancer[29] Tendonitis[30] Psychiatric risk[31] Dementia[32]
Trazodone	Desyrel Oleptro	Depression	Short-term memory impairment[33] Equilibrium problems[33] Priapism[34]
Zolpidem	Ambien	Insomnia	Alzheimer's Disease[35]

—THE FACTS—

- Long-term risks with many common drugs like the ones above are poorly understood, and there are few incentives in our system to understand them better.

- Many of these long-term drugs control lab-measured indicators that have not been proven to have any effect on mortality.

—THE PATH OF WISDOM—

- Exhaust all paths to natural solutions before you agree to go on long-term medications.

- Diligently seek to learn the long-term risks of specific medications, and then make an informed decision.

- Understand that the risks of many medications remain undocumented.

CHAPTER 5

HIGH-TECH IMAGING AND

MEDICAL MISADVENTURES

The science of imaging the human body has advanced by leaps and bounds in the last generation. It was only in 1972 that computed tomography (CT) scans began to replace flat plate X-rays with new levels of sophistication. Magnetic resonance images (MRIs) were introduced in 1974. Positron emission tomography (PET scans) followed in 1977.

All of these have become household words, familiar to all of us, with references to these diagnostics frequently showing up in church prayer requests.

They have brought much good to medicine, principally in confirming diagnoses intuited by physicians or indicated by simpler tests. They have also become a common way you can become involved in medical misadventures, ranking just behind becoming a permanent patient.

ADVENTURES IN INCIDENTALOMAS

A colleague of mine had a CT scan of his heart to see how a new valve was functioning. It was doing quite well, thank you. The scan reached down to his abdomen, including his kidneys. There was a 4 cm mass near the ureter on one of his kidneys. As soon as I heard about it, I looked up the commentary on this finding. It's common. Abnormal spots on the lungs, the liver, the kidneys, and the adrenal glands that sit atop the kidney are common *incidentalomas*, the slang term physicians give to imaging findings that pop up but have nothing to do with the original intent of the exams. My friend's surgeon said that biopsying it was not an option (I believe that's mostly true; it's very difficult), that it had a significant chance of being invasive cancer given its size and shape (I believe that's not true; see evidence below), and that the kidney had to come out. (This would be true only as an extension of the previous faulty premise.) He cited excellent five-year survival rates for kidney cancer caught before it metastasized and suggested no further treatment would be necessary.

When my friend told me this news, I thought, oh boy, this is going to be a classic illustration of two opposing approaches to possible cancer and to incidentalomas.

One school says dying of kidney cancer is much worse than having one kidney. If it *might* be cancer, it has to come out.

The other school says weigh the risks of the surgery, the risks in the future, the likelihood that it is cancer, the more remote likelihood that it is invasive cancer, and wait to see if it grows.

I looked up best estimates—easy to find—that an asymptomatic kidney incidentaloma in an otherwise healthy fifty-year-old man would be a lethal cancer. It was 0.5%.

In the end, the kidney came out. The pathology report said the cells were "abnormal." Pathology reports are often less than definitive. That's another topic we cover in chapter 7. Both parties went away satisfied—surgeon and patient. I knew better than to bring it up again with my friend. Once the c-word is mentioned, the era of rational thinking is over.

The incident is typical of hundreds that occur every day in the US. Imaging brings facts that you may not want to know, and treatment brings things that you may never have anticipated—life-changing things. Choosing treatment can become a question of fear versus wisdom.

SCARED BY A SHADOW

When I was in my early forties, I had a bad case of bronchitis with lingering lung crackles heard through a stethoscope. My doctor ordered a simple chest X-ray to rule out residual pneumonia.

To this day, I remember vividly what happened next. I had just jumped out of a cab with my wife at an airport when the doctor called on my cell phone. "There's this good-sized lesion on your left lung," he said. "Hard to tell what it is. Have you been anywhere where there might be fungal infections? Otherwise, we have to look into this." Fear gripped me, and I slumped into a chair in the ticketing area, sure I was going to die.

After more rational discussion, though, we decided to wait and see if it grew. Thirty-plus years later, I'm still here and the spot is not.

HIGH-TECH IMAGING AND UNCERTAINTY

One of my favorite medical authors, Dr. Gil Welch, points out that people, particularly Americans, hate uncertainties. But medicine is all about uncertainties. Often, he says, it's better to do nothing in today's supercharged high-tech medical environment. An example from Gil:

> We feel trapped by incidental findings. We feel obligated to evaluate them even as we worry that doing so is really not in the patients' best interests. We also know they lead to more invasive procedures. … In fact, the chance of dying from the liver biopsy needed to evaluate an incidentaloma there (about one to two per thousand) is on the same order of magnitude as the estimated chance that the incidentaloma is invasive cancer.[1]

The following chart shows why so many people are caught in the imaging misadventure drama every year. If an unexpected shadow on a scan happens to you, take a deep breath before you do anything. The chart below may help you be in the proper skeptical frame of mind when you speak to a specialist about the finding.

Chance that an incidentaloma represents a lethal cancer for a typical fifty-year-old[2]

Organ	Proportion of people with an incidentaloma on ct scan (a)	Ten-year risk of cancer death (b)	Chance that the incidentaloma is a lethal cancer (highest possible) (c=b/a)	Chance that the incidentaloma is not a lethal cancer (d=1-c)
Lung (smokers)	50%	1.8%	3.6%	96.4%
Kidney	15%	0.1%	0.7%	99.3%
Lung (never smokers)	23%	0.05%	0.2%	99.8%
Liver	15%	0.08%	0.5%	99.5%
Thyroid (by ultrasound)	67%	0.005%	<0.01%	>99.99%

Some might raise the question of whether an incidentaloma might lead to death in a period longer than ten years. But even if you used a twenty-year time frame (and again with the exception of lung nodules in smokers), it would still be less than 1% of these incidentalomas that would be expected to metastasize into lethal cancers.

SCANS GET MORE AND MORE INVASIVE

Nor are the risks from exploratory imaging limited to incidentalomas. The scans themselves have risks too: the familiar cumulative radiation risk for X-rays, CT scans, and fluoroscopy; the heightened risks for more invasive intervention to follow; and the invasive procedures that accompany fluoroscopic X-rays.

Scans also carry risks from the frequent use of contrast material. In the US, some 15 million CT exams a year, half of all CTs, use injected contrast material. Adverse reactions, ranging from mild allergic reactions to life-threatening anaphylaxis, occur 5 to 12% of the time for the highly iodinated CT contrast agents and 1 to 3% for the newer non-iodine agents.[3]

If you have reduced kidney function, I think you should be reluctant to accept contrast material in your CT scan. In other cases, always ask which type of contrast material is being used, low or high iodine. Also ask if the enhanced visibility has a vital medical reason or is a radiologist preference. Contrast material in a scan can be a nearly perfect example of unjustified risk.

I have also uncovered an unpublicized risk to MRI patients that radiologists are worried about. This risk could reach class-action suit status in coming years. Millions of people have been subjected to gadolinium-based contrast agents, such as Gadavist, manufactured by Bayer, in MRIs. Gadolinium is a heavy metal that is bound to other agents chemically in a process called chelation, so it can be processed and excreted by the kidneys. As you can imagine, gadolinium-based contrast enhances MRI readings tremendously, since the technology uses magnetic resonance to produce returns and gadolinium is a heavy metal that lights up MRI screens like a Christmas tree.

The only problem is that trace amounts of gadolinium remain in the body long after the scan. Recent findings show that gadolinium can still be detected in the brain months to years after it is injected.[4] Other patients report continued crawling sensations under their skin, and an online gadolinium support group has already been formed.[5] You would need to have a very compelling medical reason beyond radiologist convenience to want this material injected into your body.

This is far from an exhaustive list of what can go wrong with the generous use of high-tech imaging, but this much is known: it has harmed tens of thousands, killed hundreds—and sometimes made a diagnosis more exact. It has also saved lives by reversing or clarifying a diagnosis. But use it carefully and with your eyes wide open.

—THE FACTS—

- The use of high-tech imaging has skyrocketed in the past decade: CT scans have doubled; MRI scans have tripled. The less risky modalities are a different story: ultrasound is up 5% per year; conventional X-rays are flat.[6]

- Public health officials estimate at least 30% of high-tech scans are unnecessary, and cumulative radiation from scans now accounts for perhaps 2% of cancers.[7]

—THE PATH OF WISDOM—

- Ask what additional information can be obtained by moving to a high-tech scan. Will that information affect the recommendations for treatment?

- Consider carefully the pros and cons of acting on an incidental finding from a high-tech scan.

- Investigate the likelihood any incidental finding represents a serious condition, and then make a decision.

- Consider asking for an additional consultation on cells from a biopsy of an incidentaloma (see discussion of pathology uncertainties in chapter 7).

- Consider not accepting contrast materials in a CT or MRI scan unless you are convinced by the radiologist that the scan will be significantly less reliable without it.

CHAPTER 6

MASS SCREENINGS: FINDING THE

REAL RISK/BENEFIT RATIO

When it comes to health care, Americans have certain beliefs deeply ingrained in our national psyche. Here are a few of our dogmas:

- Cancer is cancer, so whenever you find it, you've got to eradicate it completely and aggressively.

- If all cancers could be detected early, our life expectancies would increase.

- If we could all afford extensive screenings, we'd be a healthier nation.

- You should always try to fix small problems before they become big ones.

Ninety-nine percent of Americans would probably agree with those assertions. I hope this chapter will illustrate that the big picture for mass screening of well people is much cloudier and more nuanced. By mass screenings we mean testing of asymptomatic people for diseases, supported by highly publicized recommendations from our government and professional associations.

Some mass screenings produce clear and significant public health benefits. The simple, noninvasive puff test for glaucoma that all optometrists and ophthalmologists use has undeniably saved the eyesight of thousands. The so-called Pap smear, used for detecting cervical cancer and precancerous cells, has also saved thousands. And yet, the big picture for other mass screenings in the US is much more complex, out of sync with other countries, and perhaps driven in part by economic motivations.

An estimated 60% of American men over age fifty are regularly being screened for prostate cancer with the prostate specific antigen blood test. Forty percent of men and women over age fifty are undergoing colonoscopies to screen for colon cancer, and 65% of women over forty are receiving mammograms to screen for breast cancer.[1] The benefits of all three of these screenings remain unclear.

One independent voice in the area of public health screening is the US Preventive Services Task Force (USPSTF). This independent panel of expert volunteers reports to Congress yearly and rates screenings on an A through D scale. Over 100 types of screenings are rated, from the A-rated ones such as the glaucoma puff test and Pap smear, to D-rated ones such as carotid artery imaging. Their website is a useful reference for understanding the many tests not covered in this chapter.

As it turns out, some of the most publicized, promoted, and expensive tests are also some of the most dubious in terms of their risk/benefit ratio. Are you willing to take a look at this aspect of health care and its potential effect on your future health?

To state the premise, cancer screening is another important way you can be harmed by American medicine today.

Could this really be true? The answer of public health researchers like Dr. Gilbert Welch is a resounding "yes." In fact, many experts in public health are concerned about this, but their voices are largely ignored, opposed by the majority. As litigation is always a consideration, doctors find themselves increasingly pressured to adhere strictly to screening guidelines, and in doing so they often substitute "one size fits all" protocols for clinical judgement.

SCREENING MORE OFTEN FINDS THE NONPROBLEM

Let me oversimplify to get us started down this road. Cancers are not found very often in mass screenings. That's a fact, says Dr. Gil Welch. Overwhelmingly, the ones that are found are small clumps of abnormal cells with low potentials to progress and metastasize. Conversely, many of the fastest growing, most lethal cancers are less likely to be found in screenings, as they are often invisible in their earliest stages but grow fast in the interval between screenings while producing symptoms.[2] Problem number two: when found in screenings, most small cancers are still treated aggressively, opening the door for a wide array of possible serious complications.

In other words, our popular understanding of cancer, fueled by the popular media, is overly simplistic. Many groups of abnormal cells aren't going anywhere and can be left alone. Is this the view of a few kooks on the internet? No, this is established medicine that all physicians know well but seldom communicate.[3]

SCREENING CARRIES RISK

The second reason screening can be harmful is that initial screenings sometimes produce inconclusive results, which may lead to even more invasive tests to establish certainty. A colonoscopy is perhaps the most dramatic example of this. We will explore this notion below.

MASS SCREENINGS FOR COLON CANCER

The US is the only developed nation where public health officials (the CDC) recommend mass screenings with colonoscopies for all symptomless and average-risk men and women aged fifty to seventy-five. Canada, alternatively, recommends fecal occult blood and DNA testing (such as Cologuard and others) beginning at age fifty and one less invasive sigmoidoscopy, a twelve-inch endoscope, done around age sixty.

Canada's death rate from colon cancer is not significantly different from that of the US.[4] And while practitioners of colonoscopies in this country have become very skilled and their procedures have a very low major complication rate, the sheer number of colonoscopies performed, 19 million procedures per year, guarantees that there will be incidences of serious problems like perforations.[5] These can lead to life-altering bowel resection surgeries, which have a significant mortality rate.

The shocking part is that in this multibillion-dollar industry, the number of lives saved is modest at best. Listen to one doctor, Robert Clare, MD, who is admittedly an outspoken critic of the current system:

> The disease I'm talking about is colon cancer and the screening test is colonoscopy. And here's how the math works out: screen 100,000 asymptomatic people to find between 40 and 45 cancers, most of which will be early stage with a decent chance for cure. That's the good news. Now here's the bad news; to save those 30 to 35 people (not every person diagnosed will survive) the test will harm upwards to 250 people, meaning that for every 1 patient who benefits, between 7 and 8 will be harmed. What kind of harm am I talking about? Diarrhea and dehydration from the bowel prep before; colon perforation, anesthesia reactions, and the occasional heart attack during; and GI bleeding and pain afterward. Of the people suffering these complications, a few will have heart attacks and die, a couple will suffer fatal anesthesia reactions, some will develop congestive heart failure, a couple will die from hemorrhage, and a few more from peritonitis complicating a perforated colon. In fact, you are more likely to have your colon perforated from the test than you are to have a cancer diagnosis by it. All told, you can expect 30 deaths per 100,000 colonoscopies performed, meaning that the death rate from

colonoscopy is roughly equal to the number of cancer deaths averted through early detection. This is the little secret that the American Cancer Society never tells you when it advises that everybody undergo a screening colonoscopy starting at age 50.[6]

Does that mean no one reading this should ever get a colonoscopy? No, but with the exception of certain situations and risk factors (such as a family history of colon cancer, a personal history of polyps, or current gastrointestinal symptoms), the best strategy for most Americans, I believe, is to adopt the Canadian guidelines discussed above and stay away from routine colonoscopies.

MASS SCREENINGS FOR BREAST CANCER

There is constant debate over the optimal frequency of screening for breast cancer in the United States. At the time of writing this, the CDC website page for "Breast Cancer Screening Recommendations" links to a table with seven different recommendations from seven different organizations. The world of mammography is in turmoil. After eight major studies in the last forty years involving half a million women, there is still no agreement on risk versus benefit.

What is clear is that there are many false positives—which cause unnecessary biopsies and emotional suffering. False positive results are quite common in the United States, says one article, with almost half of women receiving at least one positive result over ten years of annual screening.[7] Additionally, some of the small masses discovered would never progress if left untreated, but they are often treated nonetheless. The more screenings that are performed, the more women are led to undergo unnecessary surgery, chemotherapy, and radiation.

Gil Welch's take on it is this: by far the most important risk factor for breast cancer is a woman's age. Thus, the best way to consider the benefit of mammography is a function of age, as shown below.[8]

Benefits of mammography among 1,000 women
screened for ten years, the number who:

Age	Benefit (avoid a breast cancer death)	DO NOT BENEFIT
40	0.5	999.5
45	0.7	999.3
50	1.0	999.0
55	1.4	998.6
60	1.7	998.3
65	2.0	998.0
70	2.3	997.7

One reality stands out from the table: most women will not benefit from mammography. For example, about two thousand forty-year-old women need to be screened over ten years for one woman to benefit. The reason is simple: most women are not destined to get breast cancer.[9]

MASS SCREENINGS FOR PROSTATE CANCER

Similarly, the evidence of potential harm from prostate cancer screenings is beyond debate, and the benefits are unproven. Prostate cancer screening has become the third rail for the national problem of mass screening. In the past two decades, we have seen a many fold rise in prostate cancer biopsies and diagnosis. It has led to a million additional men being treated for prostate cancer, many of whom would never have died from the disease.

As with breast cancer, screening recommendations for prostate cancer vary across organizations, but the commonality is the use of a blood test for prostate specific antigen (PSA). Dr. Richard Albin, professor at the University of Arizona College of Medicine, is widely respected for his discovery of PSA in 1970. In 2014, he wrote a book entitled *The Great Prostate Hoax: How Big Medicine Hijacked the PSA Test and Caused a Public Health Disaster.* In this book, he details how our current misuse of the PSA test leads to countless unnecessary biopsies, which lead to thousands of unnecessary prostatectomies, which lead to many men experiencing incontinence and impotence. For his trouble, he was roundly condemned by urologists and their association. His book spoke painful truth to a large and anguished group of survivors of overtreatment but has otherwise been ignored by the profession.

I mentioned in the preface that, like Dr. Albin's father, my father died of prostate cancer in 1991, and I felt his death fell into the unnecessary category. Here's why: beginning with a transurethral resection of the prostate (TURP) procedure and progressing through multiple prostate biopsies, my basically healthy father was reduced to the status of an invalid with urinary pain, urgency, and incontinence. And then, to top it off, his previously encapsulated cancer (local inside the prostate) escaped the prostate and went to his lungs.

Are prostate biopsies capable of spreading cancer that would otherwise remain encapsulated? Gynecologists are reluctant to sample uterine masses because they fear spread. But urologists say there is "no evidence" that prostate biopsies spread malignancy. That's despite the fact that prostate biopsies drill an average of twelve holes in every corner of the prostate, releasing many cells into the bloodstream. There's no evidence because there have been no valid studies. Additionally, there is a small but significant risk of infection, including life-threatening sepsis after any prostate biopsy.

So if you're a male who still has a prostate (smile), proceed with caution.

My wish for everyone in our family and everyone reading this guide is that they will walk through life participating in mass screenings if they want to but recognizing that all screenings are not created equal.

—THE FACTS—

- Americans assume mass health screenings do far more good than harm. The real picture is much more complex, as our chapter demonstrates.

- Although both incidences are very small, you are just as likely to have your colon perforated in a colonoscopy as you are to have a cancer discovered.[10]

- It appears far more women have unnecessary treatment as a result of mammography than are saved by early detection of a lethal cancer.

- The PSA test was not developed to be used as a mass screening tool, and using it as such leads to unnecessary surgeries and debilitating side effects.

—THE PATH OF WISDOM—

- Consider following Canadian guidelines to protect yourself against colon cancer if you are a person of average risk. (Use one of the new noninvasive tests yearly after fifty, have one sigmoid-oscopy at sixty.)

- Remember that breast cancer screening guidelines vary greatly across different organizations and change frequently, as experts cannot agree on the risks and benefits of mammography. Consider personal risk factors (such as family history, smoking, and obesity) when deciding when and if to participate in breast cancer screening.

- If you're a man of average risk, check your PSA after forty-five, but consider having a biopsy only if your PSA reading is found to be shooting up, and not if it is creeping up or crosses the (moving target) guidelines now in effect. Always ask for a repeat PSA test before making any big decisions.

- Consider avoiding any traditional surgical procedures for benign prostatic enlargement.

—FURTHER READING—

H. Gilbert Welch MD, MPH, *Should I Be Tested for Cancer?* (Berkeley: University of California Press, 2004).

Richard J Ablin, PhD, *The Great Prostate Hoax* (New York: St Martin'sPress, 2014). Dr. Ablin dedicates his book "to the countless millions of men and their families who have suffered needlessly because of the misuse of the PSA test."

CHAPTER 7

FEAR-DRIVEN RESPONSES TO THE

POSSIBILITY OF CANCER

No book on avoiding medical harm would be complete without arming you with some nuanced facts about this insidious, most feared disease called cancer. In 2020, it was estimated that cancer would kill 606,000 people in the US, maintaining its position as a leading cause of death, second only to heart disease. People will go to incredibly painful and debilitating treatment lengths to try to overcome cancer. Fear of it drives us to try to achieve certainty that cancer will not return when, rationally speaking, such certainty may not be possible. And in the quest for certainty, we may make trade-offs we don't see unless we have medical wisdom.

THREE THINGS TO KNOW

Americans see cancer as a black-and-white issue. If your body has betrayed you by producing abnormal cells, then you need to find every last cell and destroy them before they destroy you. Right?

Unfortunately, that is not possible. We all have abnormal cells, which our immune systems are constantly searching for and destroying. Rapidly increasing numbers of abnormal cells are a failure of our body's immune system, a product of outside influences that overwhelm the body's defenses, or a combination of both. Physicians know this. They also know that once cells become aggressive and invasive, it is very hard to stop them. Despite a trillion dollars spent since President Nixon declared war on cancer in 1971, we are just now beginning to develop effective nondebilitating treatments for this multifaceted family of diseases.

Another perspective that most Americans have is that all groups of abnormal cells a pathologist might label as cancer are bound to develop into a lethal disease if not treated. In fact, sometimes that is true, but sometimes it is not.[1] Cancer is a collection of atypical cells that can proceed in many different ways at different speeds, and it may proceed nowhere at all. When going somewhere quickly, cancer will produce visible evidence in fairly short order. Finding definitive evidence of lethal cancer in microscopic quantities is an impossible task.

And treating small, stable abnormalities with guns blazing may shorten your life unnecessarily. It is well documented that chemotherapy and radiation both substantially increase your risk of developing other conditions later in life—a fact that clinicians know for certain but don't always thoroughly explain in treatment option briefings.

The third thing that you should know about cancer—doctors know it but don't share it because it is confusing—is that we sometimes do not know if a collection of unconventional cells is cancer at all. Pathologists have a very difficult job; you should sympathize with them. Cells of different tissues and organs have a huge number of varieties, and pathologists have to predict their future behavior based on simple appearance and organization (architecture). If the cells differ greatly in appearance from surrounding cells, they are more likely to be invasive cancer. If they vary in size or shape from what is expected, they are more likely to be invasive cancer. If they are caught in the act of dividing, they are more likely to be invasive cancer. If their architecture appears to be contained, they are less likely to be invasive cancer. But abnormal cells have no labels on them that say *I am lethal,* or *I am not going anywhere.*

So the pathologist has to make a call, often under pressure. Some pathology determinations are easy, but most are not. In a research trial, seven expert pathologists from major teaching hospitals were shown twenty-five specimens of prostate tissue from biopsies performed at Johns Hopkins Hospital. For thirteen of the specimens, they agreed there was no cancer, and for one specimen they all agreed there was invasive cancer present. For the remaining eleven specimens, however, the diagnosis was split.[2] No pathologist wants to miss a cancer, so there is an understandably strong incentive to lean to the side of overdiagnosis. If a group of abnormal cells is called benign when it isn't, lawsuits often ensue. If a group of abnormal cells is called cancer and it isn't, we likely come to a very different conclusion—it was successfully treated.

In the preface to this book, I chronicled a decision my wife and I made about her stage I breast cancer diagnosis in 1999. Even though we were scared, we decided to make a decision based on long-term quality of life versus a fear-based attempt to achieve certainty. We did not do chemotherapy. We were blessed to have it be the right decision. We also see that for some people, the opposite decision could be the right one.

If you get a diagnosis of possible cancer, and if it is apparently in one location (stage I), consider following this line of reasoning:

- I will first do my best to find out if multiple pathologists would call this aggressive cancer.

- I will find out if the diagnosis of cancer was made based on microscopic appearance alone or if any tumor marker tests were performed.

- I will do a whole-body scan to see if it can be found anywhere else.

- If it is not found elsewhere, I will remove it if it is operable, in the most conservative way possible (simple resection, simple lumpectomy, etc.).

- If it is not found elsewhere, I will ask for any studies on the survival rates for doing nothing versus doing a standard full regimen of chemotherapy. (There aren't many.)

- Unless a clear advantage to chemotherapy is proven, I will pursue limited local radiation, immunotherapy, watchful waiting with lifestyle modifications, and/or another conservative protocol.

- I will plan with my oncologist and family what to do if it returns.

- Are there any new trials or gene-based therapies?

  » Will chemotherapy be effective? That is, could the treatment possibly provide extra months or years with decent quality of life?

  » On a nonmedical note—I would go out and create relationship-based projects that assume my life will be over fairly soon—projects that will leave a spiritual and personal legacy I will be proud of.

  » I would enjoy my remaining days, which in my wife's case have turned out to be twenty-one years so far.

I recognize that this is delicate territory and that this scenario is idealistic. It applies only to some commonly operable solid tumors, and not to blood cancer, brain cancer, pancreatic cancer, and other forms. But perhaps it gives some perspective on how to treat cancer in a nuanced way, rather than implementing an all-out intensive search-and-destroy mission. For many cancers, these steps are not possible. But even in dire cases, I believe we need to make choices based on quality of life that go beyond the drastic choices so common in American medicine. Atul Gawande's bestseller, *Being Mortal,* has excellent insights on this. I highly recommend it. On one end of the spectrum, stage I cancer is often overtreated, leading to the unnecessary suffering of patients who would have survived their disease without such treatment. On the other end of the spectrum, stage IV cancer is also often overtreated, leading to the unnecessary suffering of patients with no chance of survival.

The good news is that your body generally does an excellent job of killing rogue cells and an even better job if you keep your immune system working well. It's also good news that our black-and-white view of cancer is wrong. And it's also good news that most of the time a suspicious image is not a lethal cancer.

—THE FACTS—

- American medicine pays inadequate attention to the risk/benefit ratio when it comes to cancer screening—and then aggressively treats many cancers that would have gone nowhere.

- American medicine takes an extremely aggressive approach to cancer treatment in most cases, including cases in which a conservative approach may be equally efficacious while offering better quality of life.

—THE PATH OF WISDOM—

- Start with considering staying away from medications that compromise your immune system and put you at higher risk of cancer.

- Eat a diet rich in natural foods, exercise, get adequate sleep, and avoid obvious sources of toxins such as smoking and excessive consumption of alcohol.

- If you encounter stage I cancer, resolve that you will consider the possible wisdom in the list in this chapter and consider saving the most debilitating treatment procedures (like chemotherapy and radiation) as a last resort.

- If you encounter advanced cancer, resolve that you will find an oncologist who will help you live out your remaining days with the highest possible quality of life.

CHAPTER 8

THE PLUMBER'S VIEW OF

HEART DISEASE

When I had a heart scare in my mid-seventies, detailed in the preface of this guide, my oldest son said, "Well Dad, at least it's your heart. They're becoming very successful now in treating heart disease—it's the happy part of medicine." In one way, he was right. But in another way, he was wrong, as I hope to explain here.

He was right because the technology is amazing—almost any heart defect is now operable: heart valves can be replaced, and hearts themselves can be transplanted.

But he was wrong because there is an underreported epidemic of overtreatment for heart conditions that leaves many Americans, rich and poor, in less healthy states than they were before treatment.

American cardiologists enjoy highly favorable press today, and many people think arteries and veins are kind of like pipes and the heart like a pump. So they "get it" about heart disease in a way they don't with other diseases.

Actually, any cardiologist will admit that your amazing circulatory system is nothing like the pipes in your house—your home water pipes do not contract and expand to keep the water pressure to your shower constant! Your plumbing will not grow new pipes to supply a new bathroom you put in! But cardiologists don't work very hard to dispel the analogy. It's good for business.

And cardiology is booming today, as America's number-one cause of death gets more and more treatable.

The technical miracles are amazing—with surgeons even fixing neonatal heart defects.

But there are ways in which today's cardiologists are using their popular advantage to overtreat patients, causing many complications and, yes, death in some cases.

Here are the brief forms of the propositions we will present in this chapter, to help prevent you from becoming an unnecessary permanent heart patient.

- The great American "heart-healthy diet" promoted on flyers and cereal boxes is partially just plain poor science.

- The connection between heart attacks and high levels of "bad" cholesterol is dubious at best.

- The huge growth in interventional cardiology is largely a waste of money and sometimes harmful. In particular, stents placed in coronary arteries do not prolong life, except those placed during heart attacks.

- The drastic heart operation that everyone knows as the "heart bypass" is hugely overused and prolongs life only in a tiny minority of cases.

- The growing subspecialties, like treatment of atrial fibrillation, are also based on inadequate data. The A-fib overtreatment situation was already looked at in chapter 3.

These are unsettling allegations. But they happen to be backed up by real but unpublicized clinical trials and written about by the distinguished physician scientists we quote here. So let's take them in order.

Some aspects of the so-called heart-healthy diet are correct. We all should eat many servings of fresh fruits and vegetables, eat whole grains, and consume much less sugar. One aspect of the so-called heart-healthy diet advice is harmful, however. The so-called Seven Countries Study, led by Dr. Ancel Keys in 1958, indicted animal fat, butter, and other saturated fats as a leading cause of heart disease.[1] That piece of poor science led to a revolution—the substitution of other kinds of fats for animal fats, the substitution of highly processed and flavored plant oils like canola oil for animal fats, and the rise of cholesterol measurement as a predictor of heart disease. That in turn led to the rise of the class of drugs called statins to lower cholesterol. More on that in a moment.

THE GREAT CHOLESTEROL HOAX

So we come to the question of coronary artery disease, heart attacks, and their causes—and whether the current view of it is correct. I started my journey in this book ready to believe that "bad cholesterol" is the proximal cause of both coronary artery disease and heart attacks, as the whole heart industry appears to espouse. I accepted that statins (the first cumulative trillion-dollar drug class in history) bring down bad cholesterol in humans, thus preventing coronary artery disease and heart attacks, and that everyone with high levels of bad cholesterol should take them. Could such an overwhelmingly logical hypothesis, believed for decades, actually be wrong?

I approached this with an open mind. Even though my "bad cholesterol" was within recommended limits, I was asked to take a statin drug by a cardiologist on the basis of a stress test finding.

I was told that statins lower "bad cholesterol" in the body, and therefore slow coronary artery disease, thus lowering your risk of heart attack.

I began investigating. It turns out that over 50% of people who have heart attacks have normal cholesterol.[2] That certainly breaks one logic chain.

True, statins lower cholesterol in your blood. What's shockingly not proven is that lowering cholesterol prevents coronary artery disease or heart attacks in any meaningful way.

In one large study of statins given to healthy men, explained by Dr. Nortin Hadler, it was found that taking statins for five years reduced a man's chances of having a fatal heart attack from 1.9% to 1.3%.[3] This of course was touted by the makers of the statin as a 32% reduction in relative risk. Hopefully you remember our discussions of relative risk in previous chapters and how relative risk becomes a powerful marketing tool. Given what is emerging about the long-term effects of statins as reported back in chapter 2, linking statins with higher incidence of type 2 diabetes, would you consider the 0.6% absolute reduction in heart attack risk a strong recommendation for statins?

I think eventually the full picture on statins will emerge from the shadows and hit the mainstream.

THE EMERGING VIEW

If cholesterol doesn't cause coronary artery disease, what does? Research on this was stifled for years by the completely uncritical adoption of the Seven Countries Study, eventually adopted by virtually every medical advisory group in the US. It said that the primary risk for heart disease was the consumption of animal and other saturated fats, as we just reported. A marbled steak or a moderate amount of bacon was a risk factor. Now, contrarian research is emerging. The newest studies point to excess sugar and inflammation as the principal risks in coronary artery disease, not saturated fats.[4]

So what causes the thousands of heart attacks in the US each year? It has been commonly believed that stable plaque causes a narrowing of your coronary arteries over time and leads not only to angina (chest pain from heart muscles deprived of enough blood) but also to heart attacks. However, it is now agreed that heart attacks are caused by inflammation-instigated unstable plaque in a large artery, not stable narrowing of the arteries over time. The unstable plaque breaks off and flows toward the heart while the body tries to form a clot around it, a process called thrombosis. Unlike stable plaque, unstable plaque puts you at great risk for a heart attack. Most heart attack victims have no prior symptoms. What causes unstable plaque? A lesion in one of the major arteries leading to the heart becomes inflamed and eventually detaches. Attempts to identify these lesions before a heart event are extraordinarily difficult.[5] So, in heart attack prevention, we are left with the simple diet-related options—avoiding foods that are inflammatory.

In the end, avoiding the number-one American killer comes down to (sigh) healthy eating, not the cholesterol-driven public health drive that has obfuscated the field for four decades now, according to our distinguished authors.

AGGRESSIVE INTERVENTIONS

Let's now move to the real growth area in the heart industry, interventional cardiology. A whole library of books and journal articles is devoted to the rising debates about interventional cardiology. I will quote from one, *Broken Hearts: The Tangled History of Cardiac Care* by David S. Jones, professor of the Culture of Medicine at Harvard:

> Methodological challenges, competing priorities, and an enduring faith that the benefits of cardiac intervention always justifies their risks have left doctors uncertain about the dangers of (procedural) complications, and patients surprised when complications occur. This is a fundamental problem. When doctors devote more energy to proving that treatments work than they do to ascertaining complications, they produce an asymmetrical knowledge base, one with better knowledge of efficacy than of safety. The asymmetry introduces a bias

in favor of medical intervention. If doctors and patients know more about benefits than risks, then the calculus of risk and benefit always favor with proceeding with the treatment. ... The history of cerebral complications with heart bypasses explains why the adverse effects of medical treatments are so difficult to study and so easy to explain away.

I have already written in the preface of this guide about the excesses of some of today's interventional cardiology practitioners, who really believe in what they are doing but have not demonstrated any decline in mortality from the placement of millions of stents. In fact, even the popular press has picked up on this.[6] David Epstein's article in the *Atlantic* (see endnote 6) is a great place to start. The article makes a strong case that it would be wise to keep these devices—stents that can never be removed and require patients to take blood thinners after they are placed—out of your body except in special cases.

Of the many clinical studies I reviewed on the topic, only one took the time to consider the conservative, noninterventional possibilities that might play into a decision to use a stent. These include risk factors like the probability of restenosis around the stent, requiring yet another intervention, or the upside possibility of the heart creating its own new capillaries to supply extra blood to the muscles that are starved. This is an amazing process, known as angiogenesis, in which your body grows new capillaries to resupply an area that has less blood than it needs long-term.

If you are having a serious heart attack, the almost universal advice is a balloon angioplasty or stent procedure. It's often lifesaving. But for treatment of partial blockages or prevention of a heart attack, the science on this highly invasive procedure is just not there.

The interventional cardiologists' view of heart catheterization and stent placement has gotten so favorable and so simplistic that they sometimes miss the fact that coronary arteries can contract and spasm during angiography and produce what looks look like a blockage on the fluoroscope, leading to unnecessary stent placement.[7] This is outrageously harmful medicine.

Then there is the heart bypass operation—the story that opened this guide, known to the profession as revascularization or coronary artery bypass graft (CABG). This operation, sometimes characterized as the best of American medicine, has declined in frequency from its peak in the 90s, but it is still practiced on over 200,000 patients per year in America. It is such a part of American medical lore that one hesitates to say anything even mildly critical of it. If it were a political candidate running against conservative heart treatment, it would win in a land-slide. But here's what Dr. Nortin Hadler, professor of Medicine at the University of North Carolina at Chapel Hill, says:[8]

> CABGs should have been relegated to the archives fifteen years ago, but they have not been ... the cardiovascular surgery community continues to announce a demonstrated 20% improvement in survival benefit (a 20-year-old study) but seldom the fact that the benefit pertains only to the 3% of all heart patients with special left artery blockages. The surgical community does little to forewarn us of the demonstrated downside of these procedures: the anguish of the multiple cardiac catheterizations required before surgery; the painful and difficult chal-lenges of healing and recovery; the 2-8% who die on the table or in the post-operative period; the 50% who suffer emotional distress, mainly depression, in the first six months; the 40% who still have memory loss at a year; and the alarming number (depending on their level of activity before the CABG) who never return to the workforce or describe themselves again as well and enjoying life. For some, dementia is the only clinically important result of having their coronary artery anatomy successfully rearranged. For none is the likelihood of survival improved.

In reply to such criticism, the cardiovascular surgical community replies that the CABG technique has been refined since the old trials. Patients are doing so well, surgeons claim, that there is no need to repeat the three now-dated classic trials that compare surgery with medical therapy.

I would sum up this excursion into the evaluation of aggressive interventional cardiology by just saying to our family and friends: be careful, get the facts, and understand today's huge bias toward action. My own story, detailed in the preface of this book, may be instructive. If a cardiologist says to you, "In view of what you've told me about your lack of exercise and your cholesterol score, we need to do heart angiography on you," consider saying no thank you. You need to find someone who will think more conservatively and start with a simple noninvasive test—like a stress test on a treadmill, combined with an EKG and a simple sonogram of the heart, called an echocardiogram, for instance.

In summary, we should all celebrate the leadership of American cardiologists and surgeons in treating advanced heart disease. But some heart treatments today fall into what Dr. Hadler, tongue in cheek, calls "type II medical malpractice"—the act of doing something to you very well that you did not need in the first place![9] Especially if you are a middle-aged male, you are vulnerable to becoming a heart patient for reasons that are not medically valid. I hope all of you will escape that fate.

—THE FACTS—

- The cholesterol hypothesis of cardiovascular disease, which has been dominant for the last fifty years, is emerging as just plain wrong.

- Interventional cardiology in America is hugely overused, often ineffective, and dangerous for patients.

- Heart attacks are only peripherally connected to stable coronary artery disease and remain unpredictable.

—THE PATH OF WISDOM—

- Eat a diet rich in fruits and vegetables and other real foods. Moderate amounts of animal fats and olive oil are fine.

- Avoid processed vegetable oils.

- Try to not eat excess sugar that doesn't occur naturally.

- Exercise your heart to over 70% of its top rate three times a week for at least twenty minutes.

- Consider doing only noninvasive heart testing, with rare and convincing exceptions.

- Consider not taking statins. In ten years, they will be highly controversial, I believe.

- Consider avoiding a heart stent unless you are having a heart attack.

CHAPTER 9

HOSPITAL AGGRESSIVE MEDICINE

AND RAMPANT MISTAKES

Going to the hospital for something other than childbirth or a routine test is a serious event for anyone. The good news is that if you do get hospitalized, you will benefit from the amazing advances in medicine that have occurred over the past twenty years. The bad news is that you will enter a system, whether in a big teaching hospital or a small community one, that is struggling with what the profession calls adverse events. The Inspector General's Office at the Department of Health and Human Services describes an *adverse event* as harm to a patient as a result of medical care. In a million-patient study of Medicare beneficiaries discharged from US hospitals, the IG's Office found 13% experienced an adverse event resulting in their four most serious categories of patient harm. "And an estimated 1.5% experienced an event that contributed to their death, which projects to 15,000 patients in a single month."[1]

The most distinguished and believable crusader for hospital safety today, Dr. Martin Makary of Johns Hopkins School of Medicine, has raised his estimate to 150,000 unnecessary deaths per year in American hospitals. And this is a conservative figure, he says.

Imagine what would happen if just one hundredth of that total, 1,500 deaths, occurred in the domestic airline industry each year. Would you take a flight to California if you knew 1,500 people died last year in airplane crashes?

Going to the hospital is a serious event because of the risks and also because you do not go to the hospital for trivial complaints. With the exception of the maternity ward and certain outpatient or low-risk elective procedures, you are likely to be concerned about your condition, concerned about the risks, and turning to prayer for comfort and protection.

This chapter is not intended to indict the caring and highly trained professionals in charge of your care at a hospital but to inform you about the undeniable risks and give you a strategy for reducing them. But first a little more background.

OVERVIEW

There are approximately 5,500 hospitals in the United States, almost 90% of which are community hospitals that account for 90% of the 36 million hospital admissions every year. Some 430 hospitals are designated as academic medical centers and are committed to a triple mission of education for doctors, patient care, and research.[2] Many of our family members live near what is arguably one of the world's top medical institutions, New York Presbyterian Hospital in Manhattan. New York Presbyterian had revenues of over $9.4 billion in 2020, and its CEO earns more than $10 million per year. I have spent time walking those halls in family emergencies, amazed at the labyrinth of corridors and departments. Surely America's biggest hospitals rival our largest manufacturing facilities in complexity. But unlike factories, they are human-decision intensive and highly prone to error.

Hospital safety is not a new topic. In 1999, the Institute of Medicine issued a report (actually based on then fifteen-year-old data) that attributed between 44,000 and 98,000 deaths per year in America to hospital mistakes. That is the equivalent of a jumbo jet crashing every day in the US, the report said, in boldface headlines.[3]

Since that blockbuster report, twenty years have passed, and laudable progress has been made in preventing the simplest of mistakes, like performing the wrong procedures or treating the wrong patient or wrong side of the body, etc. Many hospitals have adopted safe surgery programs.

Yet despite these publicized programs, despite more than ten scholarly and popular books on this topic listed in this guide, and despite countless journal articles about many aspects of the problem, unnecessary deaths in hospitals have grown relentlessly.

Why is this true? So many more invasive procedures, so many new potent drugs, so much more imaging, so much more surgery (double the rate in most other countries), and so many more aggressive protocols have overwhelmed the scattered safety efforts. The safety protocols have few enforcement modalities, and hospital deaths have continued to rise. It's not all the hospitals' fault: Americans are biased toward intervention and elective procedures. They want the best, even in a field where less can be more. And to their credit, some hospitals have made great strides in patient safety. The American Society for Health Care Risk Management gives out a Patient Safety Award each year. In 2020, it went to a unit of Johns Hopkins Medicine. In 2019, it went to the Adventist Health System. The Patient Safety Movement (patientsafety-movement.org) as of this writing has 4,793 hospitals across forty-eight countries committed to zero unnecessary patient harm. (The total number of hospitals in the world is estimated at 164,500.)

But, as reformers like Dr. Makary of Johns Hopkins have continued to discover, few preventable deaths are actually reported as such.

The affluent people I know make a comforting assumption: they assume that the death rates are higher in community hospitals than in academic centers and take pride in being able to gain admission into one of the renowned centers. They are dead wrong. In fact, they risk being both dead and wrong at the same time.

Dr. Robert Wachter bursts that bubble in his book *Internal Bleeding* through comparison studies. He then tells ten highly mediagenic stories, pointing out that all of them took place at teaching hospitals. Here's one of his stories:

Dr. Don Berwick, the Boston pediatrician who has emerged as another one of the nation's most passionate spokesmen for health care quality, speaks eloquently of his wife Ann's harrowing string of hospitalizations for an obscure progressive neurological illness. Berwick took her to some of America's greatest teaching hospitals, where, as the wife of a famous physician and patient safety advocate, she was greeted as a super VIP. You can be sure that everybody treating Ann felt they were under a microscope. But here's Dr. Berwick's account of his wife's harrowing hospitalization:

The errors were not rare, they were the norm. During our admission, the neurologist told us in the morning, "By no means should you be getting anticholinergic agents (a medication that can cause neurological and muscle changes)," and a medication with profound anticholinergic side effects was given that afternoon. The attending neurologist in another admission told us by phone that a crucial and potentially toxic drug should be started immediately. He said, "Time is of the essence." That was on Thursday morning at 10:00 am. The first dose was given sixty hours later—Saturday night at 10:00 pm. Nothing I could do, nothing I did, nothing I could think of, made any difference. It nearly drove me mad. Colace (a stool softener) was discontinued by physician's order on day one and was nonetheless brought by the nurse every single evening throughout a 14-day admission. Ann was supposed to receive five intravenous doses of a very toxic chemotherapy agent. But dose #3 was labeled "dose #2."

For half a day, no record could be found that the #2 dose had ever been given, even though I had watched it drip in myself. I tell you from my personal observation, no day passed, not one, without a medication error.[4]

The possibilities for harm are endless; there are zero hospitals that don't have fatal adverse events every year. The estimate is that every patient will have some mistake made on his or her behalf. Some will be trivial, some will be easily fixable, some will be serious, and some will change their lives forever, like the incident recounted by Joe and Teresa Graedon in their book.

M. described the sad consequences of a mistake during her husband's carotid artery surgery. The doctor came to tell her that the surgery had been successful, but while they were talking, her husband nearly died. It took more than twenty minutes to revive him, and he suffered severe brain damage as a result of that lengthy oxygen deprivation.

M. was initially told that her husband's heart had just stopped on its own. But once he was in rehab, she started reviewing his case with several cardiologists. They concluded that there was nothing wrong with his heart.

When she finally requested his medical records, she hired an expert to help her review it. They discovered that the anesthesiologist had removed the breathing tubes and all monitors in the operating room before her husband was moved to the recovery room. When his throat swelled shut, no one noticed. He was blue and in serious trouble when the staff began reviving him. Since his throat had swelled shut, it was nearly impossible to replace the breathing tube for the oxygen.

M.'s husband had a history of sleep apnea, so the usual procedure would have been to keep him intubated until he was fully awake. Because the anesthesiologist did not follow the appropriate protocol, this fifty-seven-year-old man has no short-term memory, can't initiate simple tasks, does not speak, and cannot be left alone.[5]

We began this book with the story of national hero Neil Armstrong and his tragic death, alone and unconscious in an Ohio hospital ICU. He never had a chance to say goodbye to his family. It was a nursing error that put him there after his heart surgery—an error that could have been prevented by an advocate in the room or a system of checks and verifications.

THE ADVOCACY PRINCIPLE

Hospitals have become aggressive places in America. Everyone means well, and there is no intent to harm of course, but the system has its own incentives to overtreat, undertake unnecessary procedures, and administer a bewildering variety of medications that often interact. Patients without advocates or a strong sense of defending themselves can be swept up in a cascade of events they might never have imagined. It seems like a daunting and impractical suggestion to find an advocate or to become one. But when top doctors start recommending it, as they have, as the only way to move the odds of a good outcome into your favor, I think you have to consider it.

It's true even for end-of-life patients in hospitals. The prestigious *Journal of the American Medical Association (JAMA)* recently released a disturbing study showing that patients with serious diseases and end-of-life issues in the hospital who had formally requested either "limited additional interventions" or "comfort measures only" were routinely treated in contravention to their stated desires.

In those two groups, 41% were admitted to the ICU and 18% received treatments such as mechanical ventilation or CPR resuscitation.[6] *JAMA* called these results "sobering." I could think of more appropriate words.

I'm sure none of these patients had anyone with them to enforce their wishes. They needed an advocate. A hospital is a place where you really need allies to help you with medical wisdom. Hospitals themselves have begun to formally recognize this, as most of them now employ designated "patients' advocates," also known as "patient liaisons" or "ombudsmen."—They are available upon request, but rarely advertised. Many patients prefer to bring their own advocates, sometimes even hiring professionals.

The "Path to Wisdom" at the end of this chapter outlines some specific actions you can take to arm yourself against the possibility of a serious adverse event during a hospitalization. I recognize that some readers will see having an advocate as an impractical suggestion, and I wish it were easier. I will work toward that end.

—THE FACTS—

- Although the estimates vary widely depending on who compiles them, at least 200,000 hospital patients die unnecessarily every year.[7]

- Approximately one out of every three operations performed in US hospitals is unnecessary, says one of our authors.[8]

- If you learn about the common mistakes in drugs and procedures and take a family member or a trained advocate with you or request one from the hospital, your chances of dying while a hospitalized patient are much less.

—THE PATH OF WISDOM—

Hospitalizations are the most difficult emergency to prepare for because they require having a plan in advance. The ideal is this: have someone who believes in the principles of this guide, has a serious (or paid) commitment to you, and agrees to be with you as often as possible should you be hospitalized. Determination, courage, and grit as well as knowledge are necessary qualities for this person.

1. Take your advocate to the hospital with you, and make it clear they have your confidence. Make sure that you and your advocate expect mistakes. There will be many.

2. Verify drugs. Ask about the reason for the drug, the dosage, and any potential interactions for every drug administered.

3. Insist on true informed consent for every procedure: benefits, risks, percent of complications, and ability to reverse adverse reactions.

4. If you don't like what you hear, say no. It's your right. That stops the parade and gets everyone's attention in a hurry.

5. Track the transitions and hand-offs that happen multiple times a day. Did all the right information get passed? Usually, it doesn't. Does the new shift know all the facts? (Recognize that you can't stop every error that occurs in the middle of the night.)

6. Get help fast if you see something you don't like. Do not be afraid to be assertive.

7. Make sure discharge instructions are clear and detailed. Get the name of the person to call if things go badly after discharge.

8. If you have a portable set of wishes for end-of-life treatment, like a do not resuscitate (DNR) order or a physician order for life-sustaining treatment (POLST) agreement, make sure it is enforced.

9. End-of-life patients should stay out of hospitals, if possible. I recognize that this may not always seem economically feasible for some. This is where compassionate alternatives like hospice can be wonderful relief for a dilemma.

A Place to Start for Good Hospital Advocacy Information

Alliance of Professional Health Care Advocates

www.advoconnection.com

CHAPTER 10

TURNING COMMON COMPLAINTS

INTO SERIOUS CONDITIONS

I have a friend in New York who kept getting sinus infections. For weeks his primary care doctor kept trying to find an antibiotic that would take care of the problem. My friend ended up with a well-known ENT specialist in New York, who suggested surgery to clean out his sinuses and remove blockages along with "permanently inflamed tissue." The recovery was very difficult and painful, and the problem was unresolved. Then another piece of bad news. His cultures came back positive for pseudomonas, usually a hospital-acquired pathogen. Topical steroids, saline washes, and IV antibiotics followed. My friend found himself too debilitated to concentrate on his work. Another surgery followed. By then, he was reading about any alternative treatments he could find. We talked about the developing research on biomes in the upper respiratory tract. It seems, just as in the gut, there are friendly bacteria in the nasal passages that help keep it healthy. My friend found the ENT specialists in his practice weren't interested.

At this writing, the drama goes on. He's functioning, but his specialists are concerned that the constant infection will eventually reach his lower respiratory tract and put him in real trouble.

A common complaint—sinus infection—had escalated into two surgeries and a life changing condition.

I'm not telling this story to indict his physicians or to say my friend made wrong decisions, but to illustrate how conditions that start out as nuisances can turn into life-changers if they escalate into "serious treatment."

STOPPING TO TAKE A HOLISTIC LOOK

Often, for something that's not initially life-threatening, it's better to stop and take a more holistic view of the condition. Is there a mind-body connection that could be contributing to the symptoms? What does alternative medicine have to offer? You always have the option of escalating to drugs and procedures later. But once you choose a surgical path, there's no turning back. Things will usually get more complicated.

Nowhere is this better illustrated than in the case of lower back pain, an affliction that knows no age, gender, or socioeconomic barriers and that causes millions of lost work hours and untold misery. This widespread, common complaint is not lost on medical opportunists, from spine surgeons all the way down to crystal energy healers.

My hero in this area, Cathryn Jakobson Ramin, wrote an extraordinary book in 2017 called *Crooked: Outwitting the Back Pain Industry and Getting on the Road to Recovery*. For over 400 pages, she chronicles her personal journey through the $100 billion back pain industry.[1]

It is a comprehensive walk through spine surgery, pain management, physical medicine, rehabilitation, physiology, physical therapy, chiropractic treatment, and specialized body work practitioners. I especially appreciated her efforts because I benefited greatly from the book. I was descending into chronic back pain, and through one particular set of daily back exercises I have staved it off.[2]

A MEDICAL CAREER INTERRUPTED

One of the most riveting stories she tells is of Dr. Jerome Groopman, chief of experimental medicine at Beth Israel Deaconess Medical Center in Boston and a faculty member at Harvard. After preparing to run the Boston Marathon, he had back pain set in. Groopman had complete faith in his own profession to deal with the pain, so he tried a microdiscectomy. Six months later, on a Sunday morning, he stood up after breakfast and collapsed from severe back and leg pain. Once again, he tried surgery; he found a surgeon in Beverly Hills who would do a lumbar fusion. It took him almost two years to recover while keeping a hospital gurney in his lab so he could lie down when he was in excruciating pain. After nineteen years of suffering, he finally met a physiatrist who showed him there was nothing anatomically wrong with his spine and assured him he could recover.[3] "You worship the volcano god of pain," James Rainville said to him, "but with hard work you can defeat him."

Incredulous at first, Groopman decided that looking at his pain differently was his only hope. He began to see that, believe it or not, his brain was the primary source of his pain, not his back. He was a victim of a mind-body connection gone out of control. After months of retraining his brain to realize that there was nothing in his back that should cause all that pain, he ended up pain free. Today he's in his sixties and retired from a distinguished medical career. He enjoys biking six days a week.

In Cathryn's book, many back sufferers find relief in different ways, but they all have in common a holistic approach involving body, mind, and spirit.

One practitioner she mentions favorably is Dr. John Sarno, now ninety years old, author of many books, including *Healing Back Pain*. She quotes Sarno on what most back pain specialists are doing wrong:

"They're thinking like mechanics. They want to find out what's wrong with the machine and fix it. They treat the symptoms. They should know better. Symptomatic treatment is not good medicine. What's going on right now is a disgrace."[4]

In his later years, Dr. Sarno put together an anthology of stories by physicians who have found his work valuable, broadening his focus beyond back pain to many common ailments.[5] He explores the chasm between the conscious and the unconscious mind where psychosomatic symptoms and ailments originate. He admits that many of his fellow doctors are skeptical. He certainly affirms that many symptoms are not psychosomatic. But his stories are impressive and well documented.

"People much prefer a diagnosis that suggests they can get better with a 'quick fix,' an injection, a medication, a manipulation, even surgery. Many patients come to see me only after they have tried all of the above," Sarno says.[6]

The physicians who become sensitive to Sarno's perspective achieve remarkable results. Some use conventional treatments but also ask whether a mind-body connection is going on that is causing this problem or contributing to it?

There is a well-known list of the most common reasons to see a doctor in the US. Understanding the mind-body connection can prevent these common complaints from being overmedicalized in at least five of the complaints:

- Headaches don't have to lead to brain scans—which potentially find anomalies present since childhood that then cascade into fear-driven treatments.

- Digestive symptoms are often related to stress, diet, posture, sedentary lifestyles, or sleep issues, but they can lead to full GI workups instead of attempts to attack the complex causes. They can result in a medical diagnosis, medications, and permanent patient status.

- Heartburn and GERD can fade away when one carefully looks at the many possible underlying causes.

- High blood pressure that was previously completely impervious to medication can dramatically improve with lifestyle factors, as it did when one spouse rehabilitated her marriage.

- Even joint pain, especially knee pain, turns out to have a mind-body component.

The bottom line to this discussion? Medically wise persons think of themselves holistically—as complex beings with body, soul, and spirit. They don't reject physical causes but also don't let purely mechanistic thinking by their doctors limit their understanding of their problem.

IT ISN'T ALWAYS WHAT IT FEELS LIKE

Chronic complaints can escalate into life-changing diagnoses and treatments. Realize, like Dr. Groopman, that what you are feeling may take you down the wrong road to an inaccurate conclusion. He thought his back was vulnerable and permanently damaged. It wasn't.

I close this chapter by admitting that I have a strong mind-body connection that has enabled me to produce credible symptoms of many diseases over my lifetime. I have gotten several unfortunate doctors to play along with my convincing symptoms.

In one particularly unusual incident, pelvic pain gripped me for several weeks when I was in my forties. It was excruciating. I remember one night when I slept not a wink with pain at an eight or nine on a scale of ten. We were smart enough not to go to an emergency room because there were no other symptoms: no fever, no GI symptoms, and no vital sign deterioration. In retrospect, it could have been a dissecting aneurysm, I suppose, but it was an unusual spot for that. Because the pain moved around but often seemed to feel like I had a golf ball in my rectum, I got an emergency appointment with a lower GI specialist. On scope examination, he said with a smile, "No golf ball, nothing going on here. What I think you have is pelvic pain syndrome, spasms of the muscles that hold up the pelvic floor and that's a condition connected to stress." As soon as I heard that there was a name for it and that I was not going to die, I instantly felt better. My wife, who never believed the golf ball story, smiled all the way home. By the time we got home, I joined her in laughing. The pain, once I understood it and firmly told my subconscious mind to stop tricking me, has never returned. It turns out there was apparently a huge mental component to my pain. Later I found a whole book on the topic. The young physician who wrote the foreword describes the same sensation, right down to the golf ball.[7]

That story allows us to finish these chapters on a lighter note. But the serious lesson here is to not let the inevitable common physical complaints in our lives escalate into overtreatment. Do everything you can to relieve them, but be wary of escalation into life-altering treatments.

—THE FACTS—

- We are complex tripartite creatures, with a body, soul, and spirit, created with amazing mind-body connections.

- Through their insistence on quick fixes for common complaints, Americans end up overtreated by the millions and sometimes harmed.

- Most physicians have neither the time nor the inclination to delve into mind-body connections for common conditions. But also beware of health gurus who think every condition is exclusively generated by the mind.

—THE PATH OF WISDOM—

- If you have a recurring condition that causes you pain and limits your activities that doctors cannot explain, consider if it could have a mind-body connection.

- Find a physician who demonstrates respect for mind-body connections.

- Recognize that anomalies on scans are often not connected to the source of pain. Be wary of anyone who says they always are.

- Be medically wise enough to understand when your physician is recommending only symptomatic treatment or potentially harmful treatment.

PART III

NEW WAYS OF THINKING

CHAPTER 11

MOVE FROM "SMART" TO

DISCERNING AND WISE

In the Bible, the most influential book in human history, the wisdom book of Proverbs describes three types of people: the simple (naïve), the wise, and the foolish. Many people think that these are just generic terms with generic meanings. Actually, I've come to believe they are character profiles, repeated often in Proverbs and very useful in life and in leadership.

In Proverbs, for instance, *fools* have hardened their hearts through continuous rejection of wisdom, have become out of touch with reality and sometimes even bent toward evil. Proverbs says don't reprove them or they will turn on you (Proverbs 9:8). But we often try to reason with evil as if it were mere ignorance. (This is different from being sometimes foolish, which we all are).

The *wise* man or woman, on the other hand, reveres God and has honed his or her ability to discern what is true, to start with the right framework, and to "read between the lines" in life.

The *simple* or *naïve* person is ready to believe anything that comes from a seemingly credible source and sounds internally consistent. The *simple* person, for instance, often does not start by discerning the motives of a person giving him or her advice. We've all fit into the definition of the simple person at some time in our lives. I know I have! I have also practiced *foolishness* at many times in my life. But my passion for writing this guide is that we all move over to the wisdom side when it comes to medical choices and add many days to our lives.

You see, the honest truth is that smart but undiscerning people—the simple in Proverbs—form the customer base for today's multibillion-dollar medical overtreatment industries. Don't feel bad—medically undiscerning people come from all socioeconomic classes and represent all intelligence levels. I have been in that class in the past. People who have wisdom in other areas of life can be *naïve* when it comes to medical statements delivered with great sincerity and conviction by people in white coats in whom we truly want to believe. There's only one problem. They're sometimes wrong.

For example, is it true that placing a stent in a heart artery will stop many heart attacks in their tracks and save lives? Yes, it is true. So—to extend the logic—using stents routinely to open narrowing arteries in well people will also prolong lives, right? Many members of Congress and at least one former President have stents in their heart arteries. Doesn't that add credibility?

Actually, as we have seen in a previous chapter, two major studies say it is not true at all that elective use of stents prolongs life. There are no studies that show any life extension benefit whatsoever according to peer-reviewed journals as reported in popular press articles. (See the notes to chapter 8.) Like any invasive procedure, inserting a stent includes risks, so hundreds of thousands of stents later, many individuals have been harmed, yet it seems no one has had their life extended.

How do you learn to be discerning in medical matters? How do you tell wisdom from logical-sounding but self-serving and revenue-maximizing advice? Seven questions presented in chapter 2 and summarized in appendix 2 hopefully will help you apply wisdom in specific medical situations.

Here are a few additional perspectives I hope will help you on the journey toward medical wisdom:

The crowd is wrong about most things most of the time. This principle is found in the Christian Scriptures (Matthew 7:14), and it is never truer than in medicine, where some of the most popular beliefs are dead wrong. But the wrong beliefs persist, fueled by profitability, inertia, and the notorious reluctance of medical professionals to give up cherished beliefs. Remember when stomach ulcers were caused by stress? They're actually overwhelmingly caused by *H. pylori* bacteria or overuse of NSAIDS pain relievers, it turns out. But it took a full decade to get the word out, and today there is still skepticism.

The first place to look when something goes wrong with your body is your mental, emotional, and spiritual health. You are a tripartite being—body, soul, and spirit. One of the biggest determinants of your health is the complex connection between your soul (mind, will, and emotions) and your body. And you are also an eternal being (spirit) in an "earth suit." Using symptomatic relief to treat the body only may actually lead to your demise before your time, as radical as that sounds. So soul care comes first. For people of faith, John Ortberg has written an excellent book on this topic called *Soul Keeping.*

We are not the ultimate owners of our body. If we are people of faith, we know we answer to our Creator, who designed and formed our bodies. Tragically many people of faith are careful to defend their body against various kinds of external evil, in their view, but are completely credulous when it comes to big medicine today. We operate in a medical system that has many caring and sincere practitioners but is fundamentally based on maximizing revenue, not on preserving the body's ability to heal itself. It is easy to subject our body to unwise care—destructive drugs and irreversible procedures.

We should be cautious about removing entire organs, taking pharmaceuticals excessively, or otherwise interrupting our body's amazing mechanisms. Perhaps we have not respected our own bodies (poor diet), and we look to medicine to enable us to continue disrespecting our bodies. When we are hurting or sick, we're fearful, and we just want to stop suffering. That is a real factor that clouds people's judgement. Making decisions more slowly probably sounds hard. There is an understandable impulse to find a "magic bullet" that will cure you, but a medically wise person has to resist that urge.

Today we think that many procedures in the past were barbaric, like prefrontal lobotomies. But the principle we are discussing does not allow them to be classified simply as honest mistakes perpetrated in sincere belief of their effectiveness. They may have been sincere, but such treatments were allowed to proceed out of a lack of respect for the human body as one ingenious design.

And is all medical barbarism in the past? No, there are many harmful drugs and procedures still being administered and many medical facts seldom revealed to the public.

Broken Hearts: The Tangled History of Cardiac Care, by David S. Jones, a Harvard faculty member, will keep you up at night in indignation over the flippancy with which we still undertake heart procedures. The TURP procedure, still performed by urologists and mentioned elsewhere in this guide is another example of disrespect for the body that survives today. Hysterectomies to remove simple nonmalignant fibroids, though less popular today, are still performed in the US. Gadolinium-based contrast material is still being used on children in MRIs. This is unconscionable. There are many more examples.

We're "wonderfully made"—our bodies are always trying to heal themselves. The point here is straight from chapter 2—treatments or drugs that suppress the body's natural functions should be carefully weighed for risk/benefit ratios. The largest classes of prescription drugs marketed on television in America today are not curative drugs, but symptom maskers. They cure nothing. For instance, immunosuppressants target aspects of your body's immune system that slow down the distressing symptoms of debilitating autoimmune diseases such as Crohn's disease or plaque psoriasis. They are never called immunosuppressants on TV, of course, but you can pick them out by the phrase *"may lower your body's ability to fight infection."*

Similarly, so-called "blood thinners" that suppress the amazing clotting ability built into your blood are appropriate in the emergency room to stop ischemic strokes or clear a heart attack, but if you take them prophylactically for conditions such as atrial fibrillation, you do so at your own risk. The new ones are still under patent and very profitable. But the lack of science on their absolute risk/benefit ratio is shocking.

The use of these classes of drugs is economically driven; they are not used to the same degree in other countries with publicly supported medicine and may cause serious complications. And behind their use is an unwise assumption that suppressing the body's natural healing functions is justifiable if it brings relief of symptoms.

To further develop wisdom in medical matters, keep the contrasts listed below in mind. I know these principles are much easier to talk about than to apply. They are especially hard when you are hurting. But let's see if summarizing them can help:

"Undiscerning" (the simple person in Proverbs)	*"Discerning"* (the wise person in Proverbs)
Looking for a "top doctor"	Looking for the wisest clinician, unafraid to consider conservative treatment
Getting into a "top" medical center	Choosing the safest institution and bringing an advocate
Making sure to get the latest high-tech treatment	Choosing the treatment which most allows the body to heal itself

Taking advantage of all recommended screenings	Choosing the screenings that have favorable risk/benefit ratios (many do not)
Attacking all problems early with treatment	Removing the probable cause of the problem as early as possible
Being up on all the latest medical advances and drugs	Understanding the difference between true medical breakthroughs and renamed symptomatic treatments
Treating pain with drugs as a way of life	Seeking to understand the complex causes of pain and to remove causes

Wisdom accumulates throughout life. People of faith often get wiser as they get older, and in medical matters, wisdom is more essential with age. You are faced with more difficult choices later in life. In your younger years, your body is tolerant of many less-than-ideal patterns of care. In your latter years, the cumulative patterns begin to show in your health, both positively and negatively. On the positive side, the results of a lifetime of spiritual, mental, and physical wisdom are often:

- Vitality into your senior years

- The joy of influencing your children's children

- The ability to plan for your passing with dignity

The tragedy of not having enough wisdom about medicine to protect yourself can be:

- An early death

- An early decline that prevents influencing the next generation

- Financial difficulty from medical bills

- Dying "badly" in a hospital or an ICU, isolated from family

I long for all of us to be wise in medical decisions. No family can avoid all tragedy. Our family has had at least three tragedies. But unnecessary iatrogenic tragedies are especially painful. I pray that everyone in our family can be wise, understand the medical system we live in, and partner with their doctors in wisdom even though the system is not friendly to wisdom.

The Judeo-Christian Scriptures speak to us about the benefits of having wisdom in dealing with a system that is not run for the customer's benefit:

Blessed is the man who finds wisdom
And the man who gains understanding;

For her proceeds are better than the profits of silver,
And her gain than fine gold.

She is more precious than rubies,
And all the things you may desire cannot compare with her,

Length of days is in her right hand [wow]
And in her left hand riches and honor

—PROVERBS 3:13-17

Caregivers are often compassionate, caring, and sympathetic people, but they work in a broken system. The best caregivers know this, especially nonspecialist primary care doctors. Even as they try to do their very best for you, they may not be wise in everything they tell you.

Dr. Nortin Hadler of UNC-Chapel Hill, cited earlier in this guide, says, "For those of you who aspire to a ripe old age, I place the responsibility directly on you. I ask you never to let your guard down or to relinquish your autonomy when you deal with the healthcare delivery system."[1]

Your job is to listen carefully to medical advice but look for wisdom, never surrendering your autonomy to someone else, especially someone in a white coat. Being medically wise enough to see your grandchildren grow up, God willing, is your responsibility, not your doctor's.

CHAPTER 12

MOVING FROM FIX-IT

TO PREVENT-IT

American medicine is largely fix-it medicine. That's where much of the revenue is. Yes, there have been commendable efforts to steer the medical supertanker toward preventive medicine in recent years. The medical insurance companies actually have a financial incentive to do that, so they have been leaders. There are many public service announcements for preventive medicine: "just say no to drugs," "smoking kills," "drink responsibly," "eat a good diet," "lose weight," and "work out on a regular basis." The diet industry and the fitness industry are booming.

But at its heart, American medicine gets much of its revenue from treatment and is biased toward more and more treatment, as the previous chapters have shown. More and more treatment, much of it based on alleviating symptoms, has led many of us to believe we can just live the way we want and go to the doctor to help fix what goes wrong. Actually, what goes wrong is often in our control. We are responsible to God to care for *our* bodies.

This might be our most important chapter, even though it's near the end of this guide. In previous chapters, we've said in about ten different ways that if something is wrong, be careful whose advice you take to try to fix it; it can be harmful to your future health.

THE BIG TWO

How do we move from fix-it to prevent-it early enough in life to live out a normal lifespan? It can be summarized in six words: *eat real food* and *stay physically active*.

Judy and I are seventy-eight at this writing, and we take no medications. On purpose! At our age, anything can happen, and we do not feel we are healthy because we are so smart. It is a blessing from God. But if you asked us, "What is the single most important factor in your good health?" We would both say it was the change to our diet twenty years ago, when Judy had stage I breast cancer, and our commitment to stay physically active. We all have a scary choice: to give our body the nutrition it needs and the exercise it needs or to join the ranks of Americans who develop chronic conditions before they are sixty.

REAL FOOD IS ACTUALLY DELICIOUS

What do we mean by giving your body the nutrition it needs? It means mostly eating the delicious things God created for us to consume, with all their complex enzymes, carbs, glucose, vitamins, fibers, and many other nutrients we don't even know about yet. Our current view of nutrition is very simplistic, actually, which honest nutritionists will acknowledge.

It means eating enough fruits, vegetables, grains, legumes, and sometimes meat, fish, and eggs with all the complex ingredients found in them to keep your body happy.

It means not getting most of your calories from processed foods designed to set up cravings. This is where the American food industry has had a major hand in the decline of American health. A serious charge, I understand, but well documented. Sugary cereals and chips with labels that falsely imply they are healthy are the examples everyone would agree on, but there are many foods that we think are healthy are simply not as beneficial as "real food." For example, orange juice is not bad for you, but it's not the same as a fresh orange. Not even close. Pasteurizing squeezed oranges removes the enzymes and other delicate nutrients. And taking the pulp out turns the juice into little more than flavored water with a slightly acidic pH and very little nutritional value. (Or you can go all the wrong way to zero nutritional value by buying orange-flavored beverages.) There are many foods like this that we consume on autopilot but are hard on our bodies.

So, to summarize this entire guide one more time: the secrets to living out your full natural life are just three: *eat real food, exercise,* and *don't get caught in the overdiagnosis and overtreatment spiral.*

Does eating real food mean never having a potato chip or a piece of cake? Absolutely not. You can eat desserts and even put on modest amounts of weight, and you will probably live a long time, as long as you are also eating good food and giving your body what it needs to stay healthy. We have come to believe the exception to that statement is overdosing on sugar, which is responsible for so many of the chronic conditions prevalent today, up to and including some forms of dementia.[1]

Let's do an exercise involving the grocery supermarket you know best. Imagine the floor plan of an entire store's retail space available to the public. What proportion is devoted to selling "real food" versus processed food?

You can start with the produce section—almost entirely real food. Let's be generous and add parts of the deli section and most of the meat and seafood counters. Let's give the dairy section credit for displaying two-thirds of its food directly from the source without blending, adding, or heating. But what shall we do with the bread section and the cereal aisles? That's more complex. Let's give half credit for grains simply baked and not overly processed. What about the freezer cases? Let's give only 10%—crediting the frozen veggies and organic dinners.

What percent of the store is left? At our favorite stores in Manhattan and Connecticut, 65% of the floor space might be a fair estimate. In that remaining 65%, food manufacturers promote their products by appealing to you with labels like "heart healthy" or "fat free," beating each other up and paying the premium price for shelf and end cap space. In that space lie hundreds of brands majoring in sugar and salt and highly processed food. A recent *New York Times* article explored how perhaps these foods are even designed to be addictive to the average consumer.[2] If those foods become most of your diet, you are giving your body plenty of calories but not what it really needs. What it needs is so much more complex than our current popular categories like carbs, protein, vitamins, and fiber, which we think we know so much about. We actually only know what the food industry and popular press tell us. So, a good rule of thumb is to shop the edges of your supermarket, not the middle.

Beyond the empty calories category, there are at least two other concerns with many of the processed foods on the grocery shelf.

Once concern is the use of highly processed and flavored vegetable oils in thousands of products in almost every category. I am talking about inexpensive oils from plants that aren't food: canola oil, cottonseed oil, and palm oil. Canola oil, for instance, comes from the flowering plant called the rapeseed plant. These are plants we'd never use as food. And yet these oils are not just in our snacks; they're in our cereal and even some of our bread.

This all came about when Dr. Ancel Keys released his 1958 *Seven Country Study* purporting to show that saturated fats are the main cause of heart disease.[3] (We covered this topic in two other chapters.) After that study gained traction with the FDA and the American Heart Association, manufacturers started replacing ingredients like butter and lard and beef tallow with processed vegetable oils and trans fats. The trouble is, as McDonald's found out, French fries deep fried in pure vegetable oil taste terrible. So that's when chemical additives and processing began.

As for trans fats, that drama is worth a major documentary on Netflix. They were finally banned in the US in 2018 thanks to a heroic scientist, Dr. Fred Kummerow of the University of Illinois. He found incontrovertible evidence of the role of hydrogenated oils (oils manufactured by bubbling hydrogen through natural vegetable oils) in atherosclerosis in the 1960s. He spent fifty years crusading against trans fats unsuccessfully. Then, in his mid-nineties, he sued the FDA, won, and lived to see his science vindicated! A beautiful and heroic story.[4] Trans fats are gone, but what about the effects of all those remaining processed oils in our food supply? It is controversial science, but more and more attention is being paid to the issue.

The second concern about processed foods today—beyond the empty calorie factor—is the predominance of sugar. Way back in 1972, John Yudkin wrote a book entitled *Pure, White, and Deadly*, which connected the rise in sugar and glucose use in our society to obesity, diabetes, liver disease, and heart disease. He was immediately attacked by Dr. Keys, other scientists, the sugar industry, and the rest of the processed food industry.[5]

Whatever you think of that debate, the fact remains that today almost 10% of Americans suffer from type 2 diabetes, compared with only 1% fifty years ago.[6] Astounding! Dr. Yudkin's work, like Dr. Kummerow's, languished for decades and is only today gaining some traction.

One thing is safe to say—there is a statistical correlation between the rise of processed foods in the American diet and the sharp rise of chronic conditions in middle age. True, correlation is not causality, but for me, it is strong cautionary evidence. Bad diet causes so much misery in the US today, and people just do not make the connection.[7]

I was at a board meeting in Washington DC a few months ago. After the meeting, the chair, one other board member, and I took a few minutes for dinner before my 8 p.m. Amtrak train back to New York. I was introduced to the board member's daughter-in-law-to be, a high-achieving recent college grad with an excellent job in DC.

She was just back from Fort Myers, Florida, where her dad was hospitalized for several days while they tried to retrieve bile duct stones endoscopically. She was very concerned about him—he was exactly my age and divorced, with only neighbors to care for him in a retirement village. The chairman saw I was hesitating to speak and asked what was on my mind. He knew I was working on this book. I asked her if he had ever had his gallbladder removed. She said yes, about ten years ago. I asked if he had changed his diet after that. She said not as far as she knew, then added that the doctors told him the operation would take care of his problem. When I asked if they told him that development of duct stones is a common complication after cholecystectomy unless the patient changes his or her diet, she didn't even understand the question. I quickly moved on to a brighter topic. It had never occurred to her that diet might have been behind all of the distressing troubles her dad was having.

After Judy and I started eating more real food in 2000, we discovered how delicious roasted vegetables sprinkled with olive oil can be. We try to eat two kinds of fresh fruit for breakfast every day. We are still tempted by all kinds of processed foods, but we don't major in them because we know our bodies need "real food." The key to sticking with healthy food, we found, is to train yourself to love healthy food and to dislike the food addictions the processed food industry has helped to create. We can train ourselves to find cashews and raisins more delicious and satisfying for a snack than chips, for instance. The stakes are high for healthy eating; it affects how long you live.

We also do not recommend complex diets that take over your life or veggie pills that promise top nutrition. Eat the actual veggies instead!

STAY PHYSICALLY ACTIVE

About ten years ago, a secular book made the circuit among Christian leaders. It was recommended to me by multiple friends. *Younger Next Year* by Chris Crowley and Henry Lodge, MD, is an irreverent, funny look at turning back your biological clock, at least until you get into your eighties. Dr. Lodge, who goes by Harry, is a graduate of Columbia

University Medical School, on the faculty there, and heads a twenty-three-doctor practice in New York City.

"Harry's Rules" for staying healthy and reversing aging are in the back of their book and widely quoted.[8] They focus on exercise, but he also mentions the topic we just covered—eating real food—and the mind-body connection we covered in chapter 12. Harry wants you to exercise six days a week for the rest of your life, including aerobic exercise and strength training several days per week. He wants you to spend less than you make, quit eating junk food, and major in committed relationships with people—a great list.

Exercise gets more and more important for your body and brain [9] as you get older. And you do not have to be a zealot to build it into your life. My formula is similar to theirs. Your exercise life should eventually get you to the point where you can do forty-five minutes of long slow exercise without discomfort and with your heart operating at about 60% of its maximum rate. To figure out what your maximum rate is, simply subtract your age from 220.

When I was younger, my doctor told me getting to 85% of maximum heart rate for twenty minutes three times a week would keep me in shape. I did that for years. But with aerobic exercise, the regimen you follow is not nearly as important as doing something that gets your body moving on a regular basis. Good friends of ours have adopted a goal of walking every street in our town. They end up covering three or four miles on the days that they walk, and it becomes fun. The joy of seeing things on foot as opposed to seeing them from a moving car is combined with staying fit. One of my sons loves to run and loves what running does for his outlook on life. My wife and I have covered many miles of New York City territory during the years we lived in Manhattan.

Then there is the strength-building aspect of exercise. Just a few pieces of wisdom have impressed me here. After age thirty, we begin to lose 3 to 8% of our muscle mass per decade. But we can slow that down—even reverse it. Crowley and Lodge say that seventy-seven-year-old men can double their leg strength with three months of weight training. If we don't slow the loss down and keep our muscle mass adequate and responsive, we are prone to falls later in life. Balance is one of the key things I work on to prevent falls, but I also realize that having enough muscle tone to react to a surprise step off a curb is part of staying upright. I enjoy balancing on a simple BOSU Ball to keep my inner ear in shape.

If you can invest a little time in understanding which muscle groups need to be part of regular strength training, it will pay great dividends in your life. I did notice that under Harry's Rules you don't do weight training as often as you do aerobic training. You need to exercise a muscle to its endurance limit to stimulate its growth, and then you have to give it a couple of days to recover.

FINISHING WELL

Many people think that life should get easier as you get older. But it actually requires a little more discipline every year to eat right and stay active. Some mornings it takes sheer grit just to do my "Big Three back exercises," do the exercise bike, and walk. But the alternative is worse.

It also takes a little more wisdom each year to avoid the life-short-ening medical things you are offered as your age advances. But there's a certain satisfaction when you do go to see the doctor, and the medical assistant comes in to take your vitals, first verifying your date of birth, and then sees your resting heart rate at 66 and your blood pressure at 120/80 and your weight within ten pounds of your college weight. That almost makes it all worth it. Then, even better is her assumption that there's been a data loss when she sees no regular prescriptions on your records.

If you are reading this and are far from that record—be motivated but don't be discouraged. Your body, given the right fuel and allowed to express itself in exercise, has an amazing capacity to heal.

And then you should follow that up by asking your doctor which medications you can drop. That also takes courage, but so does everything worthwhile. If you're like me, you want to be around to see your grandkids grow up, and making that happen is up to you, not your doctor.

—THE FACTS—

- Much of US medical spending is focused on treating preventable conditions.

- The enormous rise in the consumption of so-called processed foods correlates highly with the rise of so many chronic conditions in the US, versus Europe, whose citizens eat healthier.

- Eating mostly "real foods" will lengthen your life.

- Exercising relentlessly will slow down the aging process and keep you away from many chronic conditions.

—THE PATH OF WISDOM—

- Shift your diet toward "real food" while you are still young enough to escape chronic conditions.

- Find an exercise program with both aerobic and strength components to which you can look forward and are likely to continue.

CHAPTER 13

DYING WELL WHEN YOUR

TIME COMES

I was in my late forties, an age two of my sons have already attained, when I first confronted the pain and grief associated with thinking I was dying prematurely. I was consumed with fear of what it would be like and with grief over not seeing all the coming milestones in my children's lives. So I know what it feels like to think you are dying prematurely before you even understand why you were alive.

THE SPIRITUAL SIDE

Contrast my reaction at age forty-eight with grounded biblical characters like Simeon. In chapter 2 of Luke's gospel, Simeon was told why he was still alive. He was chosen to glimpse the most pivotal person in human history. Once Simeon had seen the Christ child, he was ready to die. His famous *Nunc dimittis*, Latin for "now let me depart," is one of the most moving declarations in Scripture (Luke 2:29–32).

I write about *Nunc dimittis* in my memoirs and about how comforting it is to be sure what your own life benediction is—the view of your life that allows you to depart into the next life, satisfied with the one you just completed. That question transcends all the medical questions about dying. To have the assurance that you have fulfilled your life mission—that you have done your best to bless everyone in your family, to ask for forgiveness for everything you have broken and everyone you have hurt, to leave a spiritual legacy, and to tell your story for generations to come—what a blessing! These are the first and the most important items on a checklist for dying well.

I believe you can die well even in cases of unthinkable tragedy and premature death. You have left a record of who you were on this earth, and you die believing there's a purpose in everything and a loving God behind it all. You believe that someday we will all be reunited and that "everything sad will come untrue," as J.R.R. Tolkien liked to say. So that even in tragedy, you leave your family with that assurance.

THE MEDICAL SIDE

But this guide is not my spiritual memoir; it is about medical wisdom. On the medical side of dying there are many choices—choices that profoundly affect your experience of dying, choices that create either meaningful memories or regrets for those you leave behind.

The first background fact is that the default mode of dying in America sometimes fits the definition of dying badly—in a hospital, alone, and in pain. Another default tragic modality in America is to die with your affairs not in order, with relationships unhealed, and with the doctors in charge of your death, not you or your family. Without intentionality, your death will take that path of least resistance.

Let's expand on what it means to die with the medical profession in charge of your death.

It may mean dying in a hospital without a proper goodbye because your doctors are focused on keeping you alive at all costs, and visitors are strictly limited. It may mean dying alone in the ICU of a hospital, not because you or your loved ones planned it that way but because it was the next logical step in treatment. That, unfortunately, is sometimes the default option in America today unless you change it and tell your family and physicians what you want.

Most doctors (88% in a 2014 Stanford study[1]) say they would choose a "no-code" status for themselves if they were terminally ill, but most admit that they would tend to pursue aggressive treatment for patients facing a similar prognosis. Doctors are often pushed in that direction by family members who could not recognize the additional suffering they were putting their loved one through with no hope of recovery.

Eighty percent of Americans say they want to die at home, surrounded by family. So why will 60% of us die in a hospital, having rung up major expenses, and why will a proportion of those die in an ICU, alone and tethered to machines?[2] Within the limits of affordability, wouldn't it be better if most of us could fulfill our desires and die at home or in a compassionate hospice setting?

Over twenty years ago Dr. Ira Byock wrote a book entitled *Dying Well*, which declares that "nobody should have to die in terrible pain, and nobody should have to die alone."[3] Since he wrote those words, things have improved somewhat. The growing hospice movement has made great strides in palliative medicine, and more than 50% of Medicare patients who died last year elected hospice. The percentage of Americans who die at home is now up to 31% from 23% in 2003. The cascade of complex hospital treatments that try to extend life for someone almost sure to die soon leaves many survivors trying to make sense of what just happened. Sadly, most never do.

But we need to be sure that we say there are times when it is wise to continue treatment and assume a chance for recovery if the outcome is uncertain. This is a complex field with many honest disagreements.

Asked what he means by "die badly," Dr. Byock told Steve Kroft of CBS News, "Dying suffering. Dying connected to machines. I mean, denial of death at some point becomes a delusion, and we start acting in ways that make no sense whatsoever. And I think that's collectively what we're doing."

"Why do so many people end up dying in the hospital?" Dr. Elliott Fisher, a researcher at the Dartmouth Institute for Health Policy was asked. "It's the path of least resistance," Fisher said.

Dr. Fisher says it is more efficient for doctors to manage patients who are seriously ill in a hospital situation, and there are other incentives. Among them: most doctors get paid based on the number of patients that they see, and most hospitals get paid for the number of patients they admit.

"The way we set up the system right now, primary care physicians don't have time to spend an hour with you, or to see how you respond, if they wanted to adjust your medication," Fisher said. "So, the easiest thing for everybody upstream is to admit you to the hospital."[4]

So, as a currently well person, what can you do now to start on the path to dying well in an overaggressive medical system? Even if you are young or middle aged, you can start asking yourself questions like these: *Do I care where I die? Do I want to have a "settled home" by the time I am ready to die so I can die in a place I love? Or do I really not care that much about a physical place as long as it's near those I love? Do I want to be with my family when I die?*

Everyone's answers will be different. In my case, I have a home that we have renovated and lived in off-and-on for forty-three years. That's certainly a candidate for a place to die. But even if you know where you want to die, making it happen is a difficult process that requires real determination and an ally, like a spouse. If you die of a chronic disease you can usually make it happen, but if you die as the result of a sudden medical crisis, it can be very difficult to die well.

You may not have the opportunity, but it is a blessing to have time to say goodbye, to mend relationships, and to leave your family with your story and a sense of closure.

As I write this, we are still in a coronavirus pandemic. Thousands of Americans are not getting the chance to say goodbye to their loved ones. Some of these will be unable to say goodbye because of how fast the virus debilitates the patient, but another significant cause will be the treatment. Thousands of Americans have died on mechanical ventilators in ICUs, one of the worst ways to die.

But didn't those ventilators actually save hundreds of lives? Evidence suggests that only a minority of elderly patients on them survive, and it's a certainty that all of the patients who die while on them will die "badly" according to Dr. Byock—alone and unable to communicate. A standard guide for physicians and medical students calls the prognosis for acute respiratory distress syndrome (ARDS) patients on ventilators "poor."[5] The trauma of mechanical ventilation and the fearsome complications such as lingering cognitive dysfunction, severe depression, PTSD, and others are well known to the medical profession but were scarcely mentioned in the popular press during the height of the pandemic. Futile ventilator "care," especially for the elderly who deserve a chance to say goodbye and die in dignity is, fortunately, finally becoming an issue.[6]

So how do the average readers of this book begin to defend themselves against "dying badly"?

PROACTIVE IS BETTER

The first line of defense is to have an advance directive, a legal form that is recognized in all fifty states. Advance directives have grown in popularity over the years, thanks to efforts by the National Hospice and Palliative Care Organization (NHPCO). In an advance directive, you get to specify the care you want or don't want in a medical emergency or at the end of life. But advance directives are useful mainly for patients who are in a well-planned chronic condition. And doctors tend to treat them as *optional* unless there's an "enforcer" around to specify the patient's wishes.

A newer and more direct form of the advance directive called a physician order for life-sustaining treatment (POLST) can be activated at the beginning of medical care.

It's a multicolored single-page form that travels with you in medical situations. Physicians and hospitals increasingly pay attention to it. The drawback is that it has to be initiated during a serious illness when the patients and families are in distress.

If you wish to die at home and are able to enforce a POLST, it can be an important tool in having doctors see that you are serious about not being overtreated or resuscitated.

However, a distressing article that was mentioned back in chapter 9 just came out in the *Journal of the American Medical Association* and shows just how entrenched physician and hospital overtreatment is. In this study of 1,818 patients with a POLST, 62% had asked for "limited interventions" or comfort measures only. Among that group, 41% were admitted to the ICU, and 18% received "POLST discordant" life-sustaining treatments such as resuscitation. This is clearly a patient rights issue, the authors admit.[7] Dying well in the American hospital system is not easily achieved. It is much easier to achieve at home, as we did with my mom, who died at 101 in a first-floor bedroom we reserved for her, surrounded by her immediate family. We took extraordinary pains to make sure she was cared for at home, sharing our house with live-in caretakers, all paid for by Medicaid, and determining she would not end up in a hospital unless a fall caused intractable pain. The option is available even for families of modest means who prepare years before— assuming that the loved one has transferred any wealth to the family years before and has minimal assets.

DYING WITH PURPOSE

Bringing in the spiritual element after a sobering medical discussion, I would counsel long-term prayer that God will be merciful to you in death and allow you the leverage of final words that bless your family and make a lasting impression on them.

When Mike, my covenant friend of forty-eight years, sat dying of ALS in his home, he said to me, "I'm aware I have a big megaphone right now, and I'm going to use it to bless my family." And so, he did, in a very specific Old Testament way. I had a chance to speak of that in remarks at his funeral.

I would also counsel an education process, beginning with this guide, so that your whole family becomes a united force in helping any family member die well.

You will be glad you tackled this subject. It is one most American families avoid. It will put you in the top ranks of positive-legacy families whose influence extends for generations. Wisdom has consequences. And wisdom acted upon changes generations.

One of the most gifted preachers I have known, my friend Dr. Tom Tewell, opened and closed one of my favorite sermons at the Fifth Avenue Presbyterian Church in New York with this poem, attributed to Robert H. Smith[8]:

> The clock of life is wound but once,
> And no one has the power
> To tell just where the hands will stop,
> At late or early hour.
>
> The present only is our own.
> Live, love, toil with a will
> Place no faith in "tomorrow"
> For the clock may then be still.

—THE FACTS—

- At least 80% of Americans want to die at home, as our chapter cites.

- Dying well in America is now available to everyone who plans, even those of modest means, through hospice and Medicaid-supported home services.

- The growth of hospice care is a blessing when combined with a faith-based approach to dying.

—THE PATH OF WISDOM—

- Define what dying well means to you—spiritual peace, place, relationships, people present, messages?

- Pray that God will grant you the desires of your heart, including a *Nunc dimittis*.

- Prepare an advance directive with specific end-of-life measures you don't want. Then don't depend on third parties—enlist someone you trust to enforce it.

- When you get into serious medical situations, prepare a POLST and get an ally who promises to help you and make wise decisions with you.

- Spend time in conversation with your family to get united in advance of a health crisis. Die in certain hope of that great resurrection promised in the Christian Scriptures.

GETTING ON THE SAME PAGE WITH

YOUR DOCTOR: A CONVERSATION*

DOCTOR: Everything looks pretty good, but this is the third time you've come in here with systolic blood pressure in the high 130s, and I would be happier if you were right around 120/80.

PATIENT: So, what do you think my risks are with blood pressure in that range?

DOCTOR: Well, we know that high blood pressure is associated with heart disease and stroke, and we know that having your blood pressure at 120/80 is ideal.

PATIENT: Ideal for everyone of all ages? Doesn't everybody's pressure kind of go up with age?

DOCTOR: That's true, and it goes up substantially if you have underlying conditions like diabetes, which thankfully you don't. I don't think you're at high risk in the 130s, but I'd like to see it at ideal.

PATIENT: So, what are the ways to get it there?

DOCTOR: Well, we can try some low-dose medications—maybe an angiotensin blocker like Losartan, and if that doesn't get us the fifteen points we need, add a little diuretic to it.

PATIENT: I've heard that there are lifestyle changes you can do that can take twenty points off without drugs. In fact, I've heard from a newsletter that the Europeans don't do medications until lifestyle changes are tried first or the systolic pressure goes over 160.

DOCTOR: That's true, but at your level, medications will do it easily, reduce your risk, and you don't have to change anything. Your BMI is only slightly out of range.

PATIENT: Hmm. In general, wouldn't you like to see me eat more fresh fruits and veggies and exercise more?

DOCTOR: Of course I would, but it's important to get to an ideal blood pressure level first.

PATIENT: I've heard about side effects from these drugs. I'd like to get your full briefing on Losartan before we decide.

DOCTOR: Wow, I haven't checked the details in a while. All my patients do fine on Losartan. Let me see here—the most common side effect is respiratory infections; less common is dizziness, sleeplessness, cough, stuffy nose, and sinus problems. Of course, full disclosure: once you're on any blood pressure drug like this, you need to be cautious about alcohol. And let me know about even the over-the-counter stuff you take. And be super cautious about getting into a high exertion, high sweat, underhydrated situation. That can lower your blood pressure until you pass out. But like I said, I've never had a patient report any of this to me. I'm sure you will be fine.

PATIENT: You know, those fruits and veggies are looking really good to me! Do you have any protocols?

DOCTOR: Oh, you can find those all over the internet. Pick a reasonable one though. No kooky diets. I still recommend the Losartan.

PATIENT: You know I respect that and appreciate the advice. But have there been any studies that show how much my cardiac and stroke risk is reduced by just going from 138 to 120, say?

DOCTOR: No, I have to tell you I don't know of any studies like that. There are plenty of studies above 160/100.

PATIENT: Didn't the American Heart Association just redefine what elevated blood pressure is within the last five years?

DOCTOR: Yes, that's right. Elevated blood pressure is now anything above 120.

PATIENT: So you are saying we don't have any studies on risk reduction, but we know there are side effects to all the classes of blood pressure medications?

DOCTOR: Yes, that's true. But it stands to reason that normal blood pressure is better.

PATIENT: Say, I saw they are investigating the connection between long-term blood pressure meds and a variety of other conditions. How long would you want me to be on this?

DOCTOR: There's no outer limit. Generally, when patients start on these medications, they stay on them until something better comes along.

PATIENT: You mean for life?

DOCTOR: I guess you could say it that way.

PATIENT: Hmmm. Well, why don't we do the following? I will find a dietary protocol, and you look up the risk/benefit ratio of Losartan for slightly elevated patients, and we'll discuss it again at the next visit. Does that work?

DOCTOR: Well, it's not my preference. I'm not in the research business. And that's why we have protocols. And that's why we're gaining such good ground on heart disease, and Americans are living longer.

PATIENT: Actually, I happen to know that since 2014, American longevity has been declining and that we're ranked something like twelfth among developed countries.

DOCTOR: I can believe it. We smoke, we drink, we don't exercise, and millions of Americans don't have access to good health care like you do.

PATIENT: Well, actually, as I recall, our bad behavior like smoking is way down, and in this study, I saw there was no difference in outcomes from access to high-tech health care. It's gotta be something else. I also remember that 60% of American adults now have at least one chronic condition, I believe, and are on medications.

DOCTOR: That tracks with my patients, for sure. By the way, where do you get all this information?

PATIENT: My source is called The Medical Wisdom Project. It's a little countercultural, actually. The founders are on to the fact that we're overscreening, overdiagnosing, and overtreating today. Would you like me to bring a copy of the guide next time?

DOCTOR: No, that's OK. I read five top journals every month as a part of my continuing education. I just wanted to make sure you're not going to listen to advice that prevents you from getting good care.

PATIENT: Well, let's make this blood pressure question a test case. I also don't want to miss good care. Thanks for your best advice. Let's continue the dialogue.

DOCTOR: OK. See you next time.

An imaginary conversation—no HIPAA laws were broken by reporting this conversation! Patient is assumed to be a fifty-year-old "medically wise" male with no major medical problems. Doctor is assumed to be a caring primary care physician with a very busy practice.

THE MEDICALLY WISE

SEVEN KEY QUESTIONS

This guide advocates that practicing just three things for a long time will give you the best chance to live out your full life span in good health. Eat real food, not processed food; exercise throughout your life; and acquire enough medical wisdom to protect yourself from today's epidemic of overtreatment and iatrogenic disease.

Medical wisdom comes from knowledge of the most common ways people get caught in medical harm today, despite the best intentions of their doctors (chapters 3-10). But medical wisdom also comes from having the right analytical tools at your disposal—insightful questions. The seven medical alert questions below are more fully explained in chapter 2, but they are repeated here for quick reference. Note that a positive answer to any of these questions does not mean that you should reject the medical care being offered. It's an alert that you should gather further information before deciding what to do.

THE MEDICAL ALERT QUESTIONS

Is the primary goal of this medication or procedure to relieve a symptom? Do we know anything about the underlying cause of this symptom?
Symptomatic treatment, if clearly and honestly defined and labeled, is today's dominant modality. It carries many risks.

Is this a recommendation for treatment of indefinite length?
Over half of all Americans over fifty are on long-term medications. The risk/benefit equations are not widely known. This guide will help.

Is this condition causing me symptoms, or was it diagnosed solely through lab results?
Lab results with no symptoms usually mean one of two things—they may be valuable indicators of disease, or they can be unwise paths to permanent patienthood. It's your job to discern which.

Is this finding related to the reason for which I saw my doctor or had this test—or is it a completely incidental finding?
"Incidentalomas" from high-tech scans present us with an array of choices in which a fortunate few have been saved from serious consequences, but many have been overtreated and harmed.

Is the fear factor getting in the way of my rational decision-making process?
Fear shuts down the sober investigation process and sometimes leads to harm and regret later.

Has my personal risk of disease or an adverse event been explained to me in relative risk terms or in absolute risk terms?
Medical marketing couldn't get along without relative risk today. It's important to be able to spot a relative risk claim (chapter 2).

Do I feel pressure to make a significant medical decision on the spot?
If you feel pressured, that's a bad sign. Get another opinion. And not all second opinions are created equal.

FURTHER READING

These works from highly qualified physicians, researchers, and award-winning journalists are included here because they were helpful to me in becoming medically wise. Each author is a man or woman of courage for telling the truth as they see it. They have my gratitude for helping all of us be wise consumers of medical care.

AMERICAN MEDICINE AND IATROGENIC DISEASE

John Abramson, MD. *Overdo$ed America: The Broken Promise of American Medicine.* (New York: Harper Perennial, 2005).

Dr. Abramson, on the clinical faculty of Harvard Medical School, is so incensed that he quit his successful practice to write this book.

Donald L. Barlett and James B Steele. *Critical Condition: How Health Care in America Became Big Business and Bad Medicine.* (New York: Broadway Books, 2004).

Two Pulitzer Prize–winning journalists follow the money and tell sobering stories.

David Belk, MD and Paul Belk, PhD. *The Great American Healthcare Scam: How Kickback, Collusion and Propaganda Have Exploded Healthcare Costs in the United States.* ebook.com.

These two brothers got way into how medical pricing works and self-published many stories of practices that would have provoked legislation long ago in any other consumer industry.

Otis Webb Brawley, MD. *How We Do Harm: A Doctor Breaks Ranks about Being Sick in America.* (New York: St Martin's Press, 2011).

This is a gem by the former chief medical officer of the American Cancer Society who pulls back the curtain on overtreatment and unproven treatments.

Stephen Brill. *America's Bitter Pill. Money, Politics, Backroom Deals and the Fight to Fix Our Broken Healthcare System.* (New York: Random House, 2015).

The founder of the Yale Journalism Initiative gives valuable insights into why the American medical system is so broken.

Colin Campbell, PhD and Thomas M. Campbell II. *The China Study: Startling Implications for Diet, Weight Loss and Long-Term Health.* (Dallas: Benelli Books, 2004).

This is a weighty classic by two Cornell scientists who show how American nutritionists and American medicine just don't get it on diet.

Peter C Gotzsche. *Deadly Medicines and Organized Crime. How Big Pharma Has Corrupted Healthcare.* (Boca Raton, FL: CRC Press, 2013).

Passionate Danish researcher sees drug companies as knowing accomplices to millions of deaths.

Nortin M Hadler, MD. *The Last Well Person: How to Stay Well Despite the Health-Care System.* (Montreal: McGill-Queens University Press, 2004).

Professor at UNC-Chapel Hill Medical School writes brilliantly and scathingly of the overtreatment epidemic.

Sanjaya Kumar, MD. *Fatal Care: Survive in the US Health System.* (Minneapolis, MN: IGI Press, 2008).

Chilling hospital stories from the president and chief medical officer for Quantros, Inc. and a highly respected hospital consultant.

Jeanne Lenzer. *The Danger within Us: America's Untested, Unregulated Medical Device Industry and One Man's Battle to Survive It.* (New York: Little Brown and Co., 2017).

Award-winning journalist exposes the sometimes unprincipled greed of the medical devices industry.

Mike Magee, MD. *Code Blue: Inside America's Medical Industrial Complex.* (New York: Atlantic Monthly Press, 2019).

His wife told him to write an important book, and he did!

Martin Makary, MD. *The Price We Pay: What Broke American Health Care—And How to Fix it.* (New York: Bloomsbury Publishing, 2019).

This surgeon and professor of health policy at Johns Hopkins is probably the most effective medical reformer in America today.

Robert Pearl, MD. *Mistreated: Why We Think We're Getting Good Health Care and Why We're Usually Wrong.* (New York: Perseus Books, 2017).

The CEO of Permanente Medical is one of the best writers today on the importance of wisdom by medical consumers.

Elisabeth Rosenthal. *An American Sickness: How Healthcare Became Big Business and How You Can Take It Back.* (New York: Penguin Books, 2017).

This Harvard Medical School grad and *New York Times* reporter talks about the capture of a formerly noble enterprise.

Eric Topol. *Deep Medicine: How Artificial Intelligence Can Make Healthcare Human Again.* (New York: Basic Books, 2019).

This world-renowned cardiologist and brainy tech person also wrote *The Creative Destruction of Medicine.*

Robert M. Wachter, MD, and Kaveh G. Shojania, MD. *Internal Bleeding: The Truth behind America's Terrifying Epidemic of Medical Mistakes.* (New York: Rugged Land LLC, 2004).

Dr. Wachter, professor of medicine at UCSF, tells dozens of outrageous hospital-based incompetence stories as he makes his case.

H. Gilbert Welch, MD, Lisa M Schwartz, MD, and Steven Woloshin, MD. *Over-Diagnosed: Making People Sick in the Pursuit of Health.* (Boston: Beacon Press, 2011).

Dr. Welch's is the best book available anywhere to convince you that more testing and more treatment are not always better. I learned a lot from him.

MEDICAL SPECIALTIES

Richard J Ablin, PhD. *The Great Prostate Hoax: How Big Medicine Hijacked the PSA Test and Caused a Public Health Disaster.* (New York: St Martin's Press, 2014).

The discoverer of the prostate-specific antigen is horrified by the subsequent unnecessary destruction in men's lives.

Dale E Bredesen, MD. *The End of Alzheimer's: The First Program to Prevent and Reverse Cognitive Decline.* (New York: Penguin Random House, 2017).

A world-class neuroscientist and UCLA professor recontextualizes this supposedly incurable and hopeless disease. Brilliant and deserves popularizing to get traction.

Ira Byock, MD. *Dying Well: Peace and Possibilities at the End of Life.* (New York: Riverhead Books, 1997).

The former president of the American Academy of Hospice and Palliative Medicine nails it on how American medicine prevents us from dying well.

Vinayak Prasad, MD, MPH. *Malignant: How Bad Policy and Bad Evidence Harm People with Cancer.* (Baltimore: Johns Hopkins University Press, 2020).

Dr. Prasad convincingly explains how we incentivize the pursuit of harmful, marginal, or unproven therapies in cancer.

Cathryn Jakobson Ramin. *Crooked: Outwitting the Back Pain Industry and Getting on the Road to Recovery.* (New York: HarperCollins, 2017).

Intrepid investigative journalist and back sufferer herself brilliantly shows what works and doesn't for the most common complaint in medicine. A gem.

Stephen T. Sinatra, MD, FACC. *Reverse Heart Disease Now.* (Hoboken, NJ: John Wiley, 2007).

Former top interventional cardiologist figures out that it's all about inflammation, not about cholesterol. Brilliant, courageous, fascinating.

H. Gilbert Welch, MD, MPH. *Should I Be Tested for Cancer?* (Berkeley: University of California Press, 2004).

Former Dartmouth Medical School professor exposes the honest dilemmas and downsides of mass screening—for those wise enough to listen.

Irving Kirsch, PhD. *The Emperor's New Drugs: Exploding the Antidepressant Myth.* (New York: Perseus Books Group, 2010).

If this University of Connecticut professor emeritus is right, a multibillion-dollar industry is doing more harm than good.

John E Sarno, MD. *The Divided Mind: The Epidemic of Mindbody Disorders.* (New York: Harper Collins, 2006).

This dean of back pain gurus has turned his attention to the same principle applicable in all of medicine—we are complex creatures being treated mechanistically.

John T James, PhD. *A Sea of Broken Hearts.* (Bloomington, IN: Authorhouse, 2007).

A grieving father and scientist exposes the weak sides of today's interventional cardiology. He has helped create an exemplary patient safety movement.

David S Jones. *Broken Hearts: The Tangled History of Cardiac Care.* (Baltimore: Johns Hopkins University Press, 2013).

The Ackerman Professor of the Culture of Medicine at Harvard is not happy with the past or current cardiology situation.

David Wise, PhD and Rodney Anderson, MD. *A Headache in the Pelvis*. (Occidental, CA: National Center for Pelvic Pain, 2003).

Another example of mind-body disease widely overtreated.

POPULAR LEVEL

Chris Crowley and Henry Lodge, MD. *Younger Next Year*. (New York: Workman Publishing, 2007).

Great, funny summary of achieving a healthy lifestyle from a Harvard grad and a Columbia College of Physicians and Surgeons board-certified internist.

Atul Gawande, MD. *Being Mortal: Medicine and What Matters in the End*. (New York: Metropolitan Books, 2014).

A philosophical masterpiece on life and death and medicine's shortcomings in confronting them.

Joe and Teresa Graedon, PhD. *Top Screwups Doctors Make and How to Avoid Them*. (New York: Three Rivers Press, 2011).

A great introduction to iatrogenic disease on a popular level and right in the center of our concerns.

Harold M Silverman, PharmD. *The Pill Book*. (New York: Bantam Books, 2012).

Handy reference.

ACKNOWLEDGEMENTS

This is my first book. I wrote a master's thesis at the University of Illinois, I wrote speeches for top executives at GE for a living, I wrote many (hopefully) inspirational things for the wonderful friends of the Bowery Mission, and now I write about leadership and board governance. I'm writing memoirs for my family.

But this is my first real book—focusing on wisdom and medicine. It's both counterintuitive and countercultural, so I have had to keep the passion for the cause going when friends have been polite and changed the subject. Don't worry, I won't name you!

But my long-time executive assistant at the Bowery Mission, Julie

Ramaine, is a true believer, and so are friends Doug and Phyllis Honychurch. My sharp and patient current assistant, Jennifer Depner, knows almost every word of this book because she typed them.

I got substantial research and editorial help from Hannah McKnight, Donald Bohl, Penelope Morgan, Olivia Ericksen, and James Bair.

And I was fortunate enough to find two medical reviewers, one an anonymous medical doctor, and Jaclynn Moskow, DO, with the highly current skills to keep the science accurate. Jaclynn moves between the worlds of medical research and patient sensibilities with great ease. I also thank my own doctor of thirty years, Dan Sica, MD, for many years of first-name friendship.

I'm thankful in advance for each of the distinguished reviewers who will be willing to say something kind about the book and help steer a life toward medical wisdom.

At this point, established authors usually thank their literary agents and editorial staff at their long-time publishers. Literary agents, I'm ready to talk.

And lastly, I thank my three wise sons, Ted, Chris, Andy, and their wives, who believe in me despite all evidence to the contrary. I thank my highly supportive spouse, Judy, who gifted me with the time and space to finish the book.

To my exceptional grandkids: Ethan, Jane, Laura, Caleb, Lottie, Adam, Jonah, Cecily, Jeffrey and Lydia, this book started out just for you. I hope you all will be medically wise and more importantly, loyal followers of the one true God and his son Jesus.

NOTES

PREFACE

1. Market Data Forecast, "North America Coronary Stent Market," https://www.marketdataforecast. com/market-reports/north-america-coronary-stent-market.

2. iData Research, "Over 965,000 Angioplasties (PCIs) Are Performed Each Year in the United States," https://idataresearch.com/over-965000-angioplasties-are-performed-each-year-in-the-united-states/.

CHAPTER 1: A BROKEN SYSTEM AND A NATION
GOING BACKWARDS IN LONGEVITY

1. New York Times, July 24, 2019, p. 1, ff.

2. "How Heart Surgery May Extend Your Life," Health.com, updated Feb 2, 2021. Results from almost 10,000 patients from twenty-three clinical trials in the US and Europe showed 98.2% five-year survival rate from bypass surgery and 98.9 for angioplasty.

3. New York Times, July 24, 2019.

4. Puente, M. (2015, September 4). Year after Joan Rivers' death, what changed? *USA Today.* Retrieved March 1, 2022, from http://www.usatoday.com/story/life/2015/09/04/one-year-anniversary-joan-rivers-death-what-happened-doctors-clinic/71649424.

5. Nursing Negligence Caused Pop Artist Andy Warhol's Death. The Law Firm of Rosenberg, Minc, Falkoff, & Wolff, LLP. (2020, February 17). Retrieved March 11, 2022, from https://rmfwlaw.com/blog/nursing-negligence/nursing-negligence-caused-pop-artist-andy-warhol-s-death.

6. British Medical Journal, Martin Makary and Michael Daniel, Medical Error-the third leading cause of death in the US, May 3, 2016;353:i2139.

7. cnbc.com. (2018, February 2). Retrieved 2022.

8. Journal of Patient Safety 2013:9:p. 122–128.

9. Kohls, Global Research, Jan 17, 2018, www.globalresearch.ca.

10. Joe and Teresa Graedon, Top Screwups Doctors Make and How to Avoid Them, (New York, Three Rivers Press, 2011), p. 12–13.

11. Ira Byock, Dying Well (New York: Riverhead Books, 2014), pp. 26-34.

12. Stanford Medical School, med.stanford.edu 2014/05 "Most Physicians Would Forgo Aggressive Treatment…".

13. Atul Gawande, Being Mortal: Medicine and What Matters in the End (New York: Metropolitan Books, 2014), p. 6.

14. Barbara Starfield, "Is US Health Really the Best in the World?", *JAMA,* July 26, 2000.

15. Yang, J. (2021, September 8). *Number of health insured vs. uninsured adults in the United States from 2003 to 2020.* Statista. Retrieved 2022, from https://www.statista.com/statistics/671672/development-of-uninsured-adults-in-us-by-number/

16. *Health System Tracker*. Peterson-KFF Health System Tracker. (2022, January). Retrieved 2022, from https://www.healthsystemtracker.org/.

17. "How American Healthcare Killed My Father", Atlantic Monthly, September 2009.

CHAPTER 2: THE BASIS FOR MEDICAL WISDOM

1. Pauline Anderson, "Physicians Experience Highest Suicide Rate of Any Profession," https://www.medscape.com/viewarticle/896257.

2. *"Almost 70% of Americans Take at Least One Prescription Medication, Study Finds"* drugfree.org/drug-and-alcohol-news/ June 20, 2013.

3. John Abramson, *Overdosed America: The Broken Promise of American Medicine* (New York: HarperCollins, 2005) p. 213–14.

CHAPTER 3: GET OVER-DIAGNOSED AND
BECOME A PERMANENT PATIENT

1. H. Gilbert Welch, *Over-diagnosed: Making People Sick in the Pursuit of Health* (Boston, Beacon Press, 2011), p. xiv.

2. Buttorff, C., Ruder, T., & Bauman, M. (2017, May 26). *Multiple chronic conditions in America*. RAND Corporation. Retrieved 2022, from https://www.rand.org/pubs/tools/TL221.html.

3. Welch, p. 18.

4. Welch, p. 16–17.

5. Welch, p. 28.

6. Susan Colilla et at., "Estimates of current and future incidence and prevalence of atrial fibrillation in the U.S. adult population," https://pubmed.ncbi.nlm.nih.gov/23831166/.

7. "Immunosuppressants Market to Grow at a CAGR of 14% by 2027," https://www.prnewswire.com/news-releases/immunosuppressants-market-to-grow-at-a-cagr-of-14-by-2027-301089049.html.

8. Christine Buttorff, Teague Ruder, and Melissa Bauman, "Multiple Chronic Conditions in the United States," http://www.fightchronicdisease.org/sites/default/files/TL221_final.pdf.

CHAPTER 4: TAKING MEDICATIONS INDEFINITELY
WITHOUT KNOWLEDGE OF THEIR LONG-TERM EFFECTS

1. *Annals of the Rheumatic Diseases* 2016, July; 75(7): 131520.

2. Ibid.

3. Marcia Angell, "Drug Companies & Doctors: A Story of Corruption", *The New Review of Books*, January 15, 2009.

4. *Humira*. GoodRx. (n.d.). Retrieved 2022, from http://www.goodrx.com/humira.

5. "Adult T-cell Lymphoma Triggered by Adalimumab," *J Clin Virol*. 2013 Oct; 58(2): 494–6.

6. N. Scheinfeld, "Adalimumab: a review of side effects." *Expert Opin Drug Saf.* 2005 Jul;4(4):637–41.

7. Achilea L. Bittencourt et al, "Adult T-cell Lymphoma Triggered by Adalimumab," *J Clin Virol*. 2013 Oct; 58(2): 494-6.

8. V. A. Fonseca, "Effects of beta-blockers on glucose and lipid metabolism." *Curr Med Res Opin*. 2010 Mar;26(3):615–29.

9. Kraig K. Wasik and Andrew Michaels, "A. Acute Delirium Induced by Carvedilol: A Case Report." *Journal of Medical Cases, North America*. 2013 Oct;4(11):732–733.

10. G. Hripcsak, Suchard MA, Shea S, Chen R, You SC, Pratt N, Madigan D, Krumholz HM, Ryan PB, Schuemie MJ. "Comparison of Cardiovascular and Safety Outcomes of Chlorthalidone vs Hydrochlorothiazide to Treat Hypertension." *JAMA Intern Med*. 2020 Apr 1;180(4):542–551.

11. Howard CE, Nambi V, Jneid H, Khalid U. "Extended Duration of Dual-Antiplatelet Therapy After Percutaneous Coronary Intervention: How Long Is Too Long?" *J Am Heart Assoc.* 2019 Oct 15;8(20): e012639.

12. Stephenson AL, Wu W, Cortes D, Rochon PA. "Tendon Injury and Fluoroquinolone Use: A Systematic Review." *Drug Saf.* 2013 Sep;36(9):709–21.

13. Francis JK, Higgins E. "Permanent Peripheral Neuropathy: A Case Report on a Rare but Serious Debilitating Side-Effect of Fluoroquinolone Administration." *J Investig Med High Impact Case Rep.* 2014 Jul 27;2(3):2324709614545225.

14. Zimpfer A, Propst A, Mikuz G, Vogel W, Terracciano L, Stadlmann S. "Ciprofloxacin-induced acute liver injury: case report and review of literature." *Virchows Arch.* 2004 Jan;444(1):87–9.

15. Pavlušová M, Miklík R, Špaček R et al. "Increased dose of diuretics correlates with severity of heart failure and renal dysfunction and does not lead to reduction of mortality and rehospitalizations due to acute decompensation of heart failure; data from AHEAD registry." *Cor Vasa.* 2018;60(3): e215–e223.

16. Ballout RA, Musharrafieh U, Khattar J. "Lisinopril-associated bullous pemphigoid in an elderly woman: a case report of a rare adverse drug reaction." *Br J Clin Pharmacol.* 2018 Nov;84(11):2678–2682. doi: 10.1111/bcp.13737. Epub 2018 Aug 29.

17. Donnelly LA, Dennis JM, Coleman RL, Sattar N, Hattersley AT, Holman RR, Pearson ER. "Risk of Anemia with Metformin Use in Type 2 Diabetes: A MASTERMIND Study." *Diabetes Care.* 2020 Oct;43(10):2493–2499.

18. Doiron RC, Bona M, Nickel JC. "Possible drug-induced, vision-threatening maculopathy secondary to chronic pentosan polysulfate sodium (Elmiron®) exposure." *Can Urol Assoc J.* 2020 Feb;14(2):10–11.

19. Shiotani A, Katsumata R, Gouda K, Fukushima S, Nakato R, Murao T, Ishii M, Fujita M, Matsumoto H, Sakakibara T. "Hypergastrinemia in Long-Term Use of Proton Pump Inhibitors." *Digestion.* 2018;97(2):154–162.

20. Hsu WT, Lai CC, Wang YH, Tseng PH, Wang K, Wang CY, Chen L. "Risk of pneumonia in patients with gastroesophageal reflux disease: A population-based cohort study." *PLoS One.* 2017 Aug 24;12(8): e0183808.

21. Gomm W, von Holt K, Thomé F, Broich K, Maier W, Fink A, Doblhammer G, Haenisch B. "Association of Proton Pump Inhibitors with Risk of Dementia: A Pharmacoepidemiological Claims Data Analysis." *JAMA Neurol.* 2016 Apr;73(4):410–6.

22. Mahase E. "FDA recalls ranitidine medicines over potential cancer-causing impurity." *BMJ.* 2019 Oct 2; 367: l5832.

23. Schulz M, Biedermann P, Bock CT, Hofmann J, Choi M, Tacke F, Hanitsch LG, Mueller T. "Rituximab-Containing Treatment Regimens May Imply a Long-Term Risk for Difficult-To-Treat Chronic Hepatitis E." *Int J Environ Res Public Health.* 2020 Jan 3;17(1):341.

24. Barylski M, Nikolic D, Banach M, Toth PP, Montalto G, Rizzo M. "Statins and new-onset diabetes." *Curr Pharm Des.* 2014;20(22):3657–64. doi: 10.2174/13816128113196660678.

25. Leutner M, Matzhold C, Bellach L, Deischinger C, Harreiter J, Thurner S, Klimek P, Kautzky-Willer A. "Diagnosis of osteoporosis in statin-treated patients is dose-dependent." *Ann Rheum Dis.* 2019 Dec;78(12):1706–1711.

26. Kim SY, Kim SJ, Yoon D, Hong SW, Park S, Ock CY. "A Case of Statin-Induced Interstitial Pneumonitis due to Rosuvastatin." *Tuberc Respir Dis (Seoul).* 2015 Jul;78(3):281–5.

27. Ward FL, John R, Bargman JM, McQuillan RF. "Renal Tubular Toxicity Associated with Rosuvastatin Therapy." *Am J Kidney Dis.* 2017 Mar;69(3):473–476.

28. "LiverTox: Clinical and Research Information on Drug-Induced Liver Injury" [internet]. Bethesda (MD): National Institute of Diabetes and Digestive and Kidney Diseases; 2012-. Simvastatin.

29. Ravnskov U, McCully KS, Rosch PJ. "The statin-low cholesterol-cancer conundrum." *QJM*. 2012 Apr;105(4):383–8.

30. Esenkaya I, Unay K. "Tendon, tendon healing, hyperlipidemia and statins." *Muscles Ligaments Tendons J*. 2012 Apr 1;1(4):169–71.

31. Cham S, Koslik HJ, Golomb BA. "Mood, Personality, and Behavior Changes During Treatment with Statins: A Case Series." *Drug Saf Case Rep*. 2016 Dec;3(1):1.

32. Miller, DW. "Fallacies in modern medicine: statins and the cholesterol-heart hypothesis." *Journal of American Physicians and Surgeons*. 2015;20(2)54–57.

33. Roth AJ, McCall WV, Liguori A. "Cognitive, psychomotor and polysomnographic effects of trazodone in primary insomniacs." *J Sleep Res*. 2011 Dec;20(4):552–8.

34. Hoffmann P, Neu ET, Neu D. "Penile amputation after trazodone-induced priapism: a case report." *Prim Care Companion J Clin Psychiatry*. 2010;12(2): PCC.09l00816.

35. Cheng HT, Lin FJ, Erickson SR, Hong JL, Wu CH. "The Association Between the Use of Zolpidem and the Risk of Alzheimer's Disease Among Older People." *J Am Geriatr Soc*. 2017 Nov;65(11):2488–2495.

CHAPTER 5: HIGH TECH IMAGING AND MEDICAL MISADVENTURES

1. H. Gilbert Welch, *Over-Diagnosed: Making People Sick in the Pursuit of Health* (Boston Beacon Press, 2011), p. 93.

2. Welch, p. 95.

3. *Radiology*, 6/1/1990, p. 7.

4. FDA Drug Safety Podcast, "FDA warns that gadolinium-base contrast agents (GBCAs) are retained in the body; requires new class warnings," https://www.fda.gov/drugs/fda-drug-safety-podcasts/fda-drug-safety-podcast-fda-warns-gadolinium-based-contrast-agents-gbcas-are-retained-body-requires

5. "Symptoms associated with Gadolinium Toxicity," https://gadoliniumtoxicity.com/help/symptoms/.

6. U.S. National Library of Medicine. (n.d.). National Center for Biotechnology Information. Retrieved 2022, from https://www.ncbi.nlm.nih.gov/.

7. Public Library of Science, UK, March 15, 2019, journal-pone.0213373.

CHAPTER 6: MASS SCREENINGS: THE REAL RISK/BENEFIT RATIO

1. "Cancer Screening in the United States", Robert A. Smith, et al., A Cancer Journal for Clinicians, Volume 69, Issue 3.

2. H. Gilbert Welch, *Should I Be Tested for Cancer?* (Berkley: University of California Press, 2004), pp. 18–21.

3. Welch, *Should I Be Tested*, p. 8.

4. Sabin Russell, "At half the cost, Canadian colorectal cancer survival similar to that of U.S," https://www.fredhutch.org/en/news/center-news/2018/05/canada-us-comparison-colorectal-cancer-cost-outcomes.html.

5. iData Research, "An Astounding 19 Million Colonoscopies Are Performed Annually in the United States," https://idataresearch.com/an-astounding-19-million-colonoscopies-are-performed-annually-in-the-united-states/.

6. Robert Clare, "I'm skeptical about … screening colonoscopies," https://robertclaremd.com/im-skeptical-about-screening-colonoscopies/.

7. Talva Salz et al., "False positive mammograms in Europe: Do they affect reattendance?" https://www.ncbi.nlm.nih.gov/pmc/articles/PMC3160730/.

8. H. Gilbert Welch, *Over-Diagnosed: Making People Sick in the Pursuit of Health*, (Boston, Beacon Press, 2011) p. 28.

9. Welch, *Should I Be Tested?* pp. 34–35.

10. Clare, "I'm skeptical."

CHAPTER 7: FEAR-DRIVEN RESPONSES TO THE POSSIBILITY OF CANCER

1. H. Gilbert Welch, Should I Be Tested, p. 8.

2. Welch, *Should I Be Tested,* p. 98.

CHAPTER 8: THE PLUMBER'S VIEW OF HEART DISEASE

1. *The Seven countries study - the first epidemiological nutrition study, since 1958.* Seven Countries Study | The first study to relate diet with cardiovascular disease. (2020, February 11). Retrieved 2022, from https://www.sevencountriesstudy.com/.

2. Sachdeva, A., Cannon, C. P., Deedwania, P. C., Labresh, K. A., Smith, S. C., Dai, D., Hernandez, A., & Fonarow, G. C. (2008, October 22). *Lipid levels in patients hospitalized with coronary artery disease: An analysis of 136,905 hospitalizations in get with the guidelines.* American Heart Journal. Retrieved February 24, 2022, from https://pubmed.ncbi.nlm.nih.gov/19081406/

3. Norton M. Hadler. *The Last Well Person: How to Stay Well Despite the Healthcare System*, (London: McGill-Queen's University Press, 2013), p. 38.

4. Frank Hu, *JAMA: Internal Medicine*, 2014 quoted in *Harvard Health Publishing*, May 2017.

5. Mehta, D. A. B., & Shah, D. S. (2006, January). *Unstable or high risk plaque: How do we approach it?* Medical Journal, Armed Forces India. Retrieved 2022, from https://www.ncbi.nlm.nih.gov/pmc/articles/PMC4923293/

6. "Heart Stents are Useless for Most Stable Patients; They're Still Widely Used, " *New York Times*, February 12, 2018. David Epstein and ProPublica, "When Evidence Says No but Doctors Say Yes." *The Atlantic*, February 22, 2017. "Are Doctors Exposing Heart Patients to Unnecessary Cardiac Procedures?", *US News and World Report*, February 11, 2015.

7. "A Simple Fix to Avoid Unnecessary Coronary Stents," *Jefferson University Hospital News*, March 20, 2017.

8. Hadler, p. 23.

9. Hadler, p. 203.

CHAPTER 9: HOSPITAL AGGRESSIVE MEDICINE AND RAMPANT MISTAKES

1. "Adverse Events in Hospitals: National Incidence Among Medicare Beneficiaries Department of Health and Human Services," Office of the Inspector General, November 2010.

2. Mike Magee, *Code Blue: Inside America's Medical Industrial Complex* (New York: Atlantic Monthly Press, 2019), p.103.

3. Robert Wachter and Kaveh G. Shojania, *Internal Bleeding*, (New York: Rugged Land, 2005), p. 56.

4. Wachter and Shojania, pp. 97–98.

5. Joe and Teresa Graedon, *Top Screwups Doctors Make and How to Avoid Them* (New York: Three Rivers Press, 2011), pp. 13–14.

6. *Journal of the American Medical Association online*, Feb 16, 2020, Truog and Fried. https://jamanetwork.com.

7. Graedon, p. 12.

8. Eric Topol, *Deep Medicine*, (New York: Basic Books 2019), p. 26.

CHAPTER 10: TURNING COMMON COMPLAINTS INTO SERIOUS CONDITIONS

1. Cathryn Jakobson Ramin, Crooked: Outwitting the Back Pain Industry and Getting on the Road to Recovery, (New York: HarperCollins, 2017).

2. Ramin, p 241–42. Bio-mechanist Dr. Stuart McGill of Waterloo University in Canada has his Big Three Exercises which I practice daily.

3. Ramin, p. 248, James Rainville of New England Baptist Hospital.

4. Ramin, p.192.

5. John E Sarno, *The Divided Mind: The Epidemic of Mind/Body Disorders*, (New York: Harper, 2006).

6. Sarno, p. 32.

7. David Wise and Rodney Anderson, *A Headache in the Pelvis* (Occidental, CA: National Center for Pelvic Pain Research, 2003), p.14.

CHAPTER 11: MOVE FROM SMART TO DISCERNING AND WARY

1. Nortin M. Hadler, The Last Well Person: How to Stay Well Despite the Healthcare System, (London: McGill-Queen's University Press, 2013), p. 203.

CHAPTER 12: MOVE FROM FIX-IT TO PREVENT-IT

1. Dale Bredeson, The End of Alzheimer's, (Los Angeles, UCLA Press, 2017).

2. Anahad O'Connor, "No One Can Eat Just One, Perhaps by Design," *New York Times*, February 23, 2021, p. D-6.

3. The current consensus labels Dr. Keys's Seven Country Study as inadequate science. The study left out Denmark, France, and Norway, where the diet is rich in fats, but the occurrence of heart disease is low, and Chile, where the diet is low in fat, yet occurrence of heart disease is high. Despite that, five decades later, our heart disease industry is still based on Keys's theory.

4. Hafner, K. (2017, June 1). Fred A. Kummerow, an early opponent of trans fats, dies at 102. *New York Times*. Retrieved February 28, 2022, from https://www.nytimes.com/2017/06/01/science/fred-kummerow-dead-biochemist-ban-trans-fatty-acids.html

5. For more information on the issue, listen to "Sugar, The Bitter Truth," Robert Lustig, 2009, YouTube.

6. CDC's Division of Diabetes Translation. (2017, April). Long-term Trends in Diabetes.

7. For a good summary of the debate, see *American Society for Biochemistry and Molecular Biology Magazine*, Nov 2, 2012. Debate over omega 6 rich oils has increased since then, with American Heart Association scientists lined up against others.

8. Chris Crowley and Henry S. Lodge MD., *Younger Next Year: Live Strong, Fit and Sexy Until You're 80 and Beyond* (New York: Workman Publishing, 2007), Appendix A.

9. Brock Armstrong. "How Exercise Affects Your Brain," *Scientific American*, December 26, 2018.

CHAPTER 13: DYING WELL WHEN YOUR TIME COMES

1.   Stanford School of Medicine news release 2014/05.

2.   Stanford School of Medicine. (2013, April 21). *Where do Americans die?* Multi-cultural Palliative Care Portal. Retrieved 2022, from https://palliative.stanford.edu/home-hospice-home-care-of-the-dying-patient/where-do-americans-die/

3.   Ira Byock, *Dying Well* (New York: Penguin, 1997), p. xiv.

4.   Cross, S. H., & Warraich, H. J. (2019, December 12). *Changes in the place of death in the United States: Nejm.* New England Journal of Medicine. Retrieved February 24, 2022, from https://www.nejm.org/doi/full/10.1056/nejmc1911892

5.   Papadakas, McPhee and Rabow, *Current Medical Diagnosis and Treatment* (New York, McGraw Hill, 2019), p. 333.

6.   Wilkinson, D. J. C., &; Savulescu, J. (2011, April). Knowing when to stop: Futility in the ICU. Current opinion in anaesthesiology. Retrieved February 28, 2022, from http://www.ncbi.nlm.nih.gov/pmc/articles/PMC3252683

7.   Truog, R. D., & Fried, T. R. (2020). Physician Orders for Life-Sustaining Treatment and Limiting Overtreatment at the End of Life. *JAMA*, 323(10), 934–935. https://doi.org/10.1001/jama.2019.22522

8.   Fifth Avenue Presbyterian Church is a legacy institution for my family. My grandfather, Minot C. Morgan Jr, copastored there from 1928 to 1933 before he went on to a seventeen-year pastorate at First Presbyterian Church, Greenwich, Connecticut.

INDEX